SKULL FRAGMENTS
EXPRESSIONS OF MY TBI LIFE

LEN ROACH

◆ FriesenPress

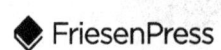

One Printers Way
Altona, MB R0G 0B0
Canada

www.friesenpress.com

Copyright © 2024 by Len Roach
First Edition — 2024

All rights reserved.

Editor: Christopher Gooding

Photographer: Sebastian Buzzalino

No part of this publication may be reproduced in any form, or by any means, electronic or mechanical, including photocopying, recording, or any information browsing, storage, or retrieval system, without permission in writing from FriesenPress.

ISBN
978-1-03-917123-7 (Hardcover)
978-1-03-917122-0 (Paperback)
978-1-03-917124-4 (eBook)

1. BIOGRAPHY & AUTOBIOGRAPHY, MEDICAL

Distributed to the trade by The Ingram Book Company

To my family and friends.
Thank you for your love and support.

To the doctors, nurses, and therapists,
I am eternally grateful.

To my fellow survivors,
May you be granted perseverance, serenity, and hope.

Introduction
A Breath before
Rambling

I am unsure to number of words into this I am as I write this obligatory introduction. After I aggressively punched my laptop, I was certain that another outburst had cost me. At least only a chapter this time; the screen faded fast before my eyes. It was a chapter about my marriage. I suppose it could be a blessing in disguise, as it was more about the marriage itself than the subject at hand.

I recall the pandemic raging away when I started, my second lockdown spawning the first deluge of words. Even now, in this very moment, I reflect on how, on this night six years ago, my life was significantly thrown askew on waves of encephalic trauma. Just over thirty years from the first time.

I would be remiss if I did not address crucial factors from the onset. The forthcoming series of anecdotes and testimonials began as a personal need to communicate about not so much my life but the lives of those that have not fared as well as me on account of their brain health.

I have no medical education or training in any way—a fact that should be evident pretty much immediately. The medical and anatomical terms I use have come to me through therapists, doctors, and personal research. I assume I use the wrong terminology often. I am not an expert on the subject; I am merely experienced.

Despite the severity of the two pivotal events to which I refer throughout, I reclaimed and retained a cognizance that exceeded expectations. I put in the work because I was able to. There are those that suffer brain injuries who are not as lucky. It was for them that I started writing. I wanted to attempt to lend a voice to my brothers and sisters who struggle to communicate the ways, both subtle and apparent, in which ABI/TBI—acquired or traumatic brain injury—have affected damn near everything.

Obviously, it wouldn't take long until my long-suppressed sigh finally escaped. As memories and thoughts wafted up from my past to clamber haphazardly on page after page, I found ever more of myself in words unadulterated. In the morning I would peruse and polish, the latter as little as needed. The language and rhythm had to be organic, a testament to my verbosity and penchant for prattling on. A plausible affliction of mild logorrhea garnered from my injuries. Honest to a fault, I cannot swear to the truthfulness of these words. Years and damage do memories no favour, so I relate events only to the best of my ability to recall them. If the tone seems by times boastful, flippant, or deprecating, I can only hope it is equally so, as that would more sincerely reflect the truth of my situation.

I shall conclude this preamble with an off-the-cuff explanation as to why I opted to leave out the names of those who were involved. Though the omission of their identity does have the reward of side stepping most possible legal trouble, this was not my primary motivation. I use primarily pronouns, with few exceptions, to illustrate the self-absorbed nature of these reflections. Those involved know who they are and my respectful gratitude for them. Furthermore, by excluding the names of the ancillary characters in my story, I make it possible for readers to regard them as anyone, in any life. And on the flip side, those that hindered, harmed, or vexed my existence don't deserve the courtesy of being identified by name.

1
"Fall in a Small Town"

It is going to be challenging, looking back with different eyes. There are many years between this night, the first of July 2020, in Calgary, Alberta, and October 8, 1991, in Pugwash, Nova Scotia.

Now a man in my early forties, I confess that it's all not as clear as it once was.

Nonetheless, let me attempt to expound the details of what life was like after my fall. Mind you, this is mostly based on what I was told well after the fact.

A friend and I were bored, restless fourteen-year-olds in an idyllic coastal town. One night, we opted to sneak out of his bedroom window to meander about town. I have no recollection of that night—nothing at all. It is the epicentre of a gap in my memory that radiates in such a way that memory before and after becoming more redacted and blackened closer they are to the point of impact, the moment I slipped and fell thirteen feet onto concrete. I was writing obscenities on a second-storey window from the vantage of an adjacent ledge. There was likely no more of a reason to be doing it than not caring enough to think of reason not to—the uninspired and underwhelming type of irrational fuckery that has be a generational condition in small towns everywhere. Nothing destructive or maliciously inspired. No booze or drugs. We were sober and simply aware of the drudgery of it all. Just looking for some shits and giggles, a senseless act to have a chuckle about. I don't remember our motivation for climbing up on the roof. I don't recall whose idea it was—it could have been mine. I also don't recall walking to hospital next door.

My memory before and after, like I said, is absent. Only blackness there, not even the faintest glow of recollection. A dark, expanse of blotted-out memory for stretches in both directions. I can recall nothing of the weeks before and nothing for a solid ten days after. That isn't entirely true. My memory after the fall does include a couple flashes of light. For example, a nurse's face in the ambulance and the fluorescent lights above my gurney clicking past my flickering eyes as my brain sought to endure. Not much more.

When I fell, I fell hard. I slid down the brick with the top of my forehead, leaving a trail of blood and bits of shoulder-length, dark brown hair. My skull connected with the concrete at the top of my eye orbit with all the tenderness of a hate-fueled sledgehammer. A compound fracture of the eye orbit was followed by a break of my nose and a smashing of notable chunks out of a couple of teeth. It was my own personal micro-dose of a near fatality. Yet, despite this visceral trauma, I was able to get up to one knee before my friend reached me. Blood was escaping with aggressive nonchalance from my mouth and nose. A pool coagulated at the point of impact, a final splash of red at the bottom of that gory tendril of blood and hair. It would remain until Monday, when school returned after a weekend of rest and raucousness alike. I was told that the stain remained until a heavy rain expunged it from the schoolyard. I cannot speak on the effect such a sight had on the students of Pugwash District High. Nor can I explain how the ghastly truth of the moment had yet to take reign.

Bloodied and bashed to shit, I started formulating a lie to cover our tracks, something about tripping over barbells. Didn't want to catch shit for sneaking out, you see.

My friend, having informed me weeks later of that obviously forgotten tidbit also told me his response to the situation at the time. Apparently, he looked at my mangled mug, then the roof, then the pool of my fresh blood simmering in moonlight and ill omens. Finally, he looked me in the eye, and said, "The hospital is closer." I agreed and we went two doors down to the emergency room of Northumberland Hospital.

A small-town hospital where babies are born and a man can get few stitches after a slip with a fish knife, they took a quick look at my shade of carnage and thought I had been in a motorcycle accident. Once they knew the facts, they immediately called my parents, waking them from sleep at 2 a.m., to tell them Lenny had fallen off the roof of the high school and they needed to get to the hospital at once. It was serious. No denying that, but no examination had occurred yet, so the extent of the severity was yet to be discerned. One obvious indicator that this was by no means run of the mill soon appeared.

By the time my parents arrived, estimated to be five to eight minutes after they received the call, the swelling had reached its crescendo. The membrane between my skull and brain had been torn, like a fissure in a dam, allowing spinal fluid to seep out and flood my cheeks. My eyes fully shut by engorged flesh, only the tip of my nose could be seen. It was a sight so unimaginable that my older brother needed a wheelchair upon encountering it. The shock of seeing me drained him of the vitality to stand. The panic and fear were all-engulfing. The swelling would remain for days. I'm glad I cannot recall those days. I don't need to live with the memory of the chaos around me as I struggled blindly to cope with a brain in utter turmoil. I don't want to know. I just know it was too much for a coastal village hospital because I was transported post haste to

Amherst. The hospital there was more equipped for such emergencies. My parents would drive me as it was faster than waiting for the ambulance.

Nothing is a direct memory when it comes to the four of five days while I was in Amherst General. It was the larger hospital in the county, as Amherst itself was the capital. There is no personal, subjective record of that time. What I was thinking, how I felt are unknown. There exists a chasm of nothingness, skirted by distant banks of cognizance. I have no memory of tears or pain, confusion or fear. Only the smile of a nurse and those fluorescent lights remain. I know that it was during this time that the swelling subsided enough that I could open my eyes, but I can't bring to light what I saw when I did. A probable mix of medication and trauma had left my brain too limp and fragile to grasp or retain anything. My frontal lobe was in panic mode as my cerebral cortex careened into desperately frantic synaptic misfires. No recollection. Somewhere in my skull a kill switch had been pressed, denying me access to the cognitive faculty of memory.

My family was there: my mother and father, my brother and younger sister. So was the uncertainty in all its forms, lingering around their minds as the doctors and nurses came and went. They stayed with me, my family, until Sunday night. My siblings had school Monday morning, and I believe my dad had to work. Sunday night it was time for my dad to explain that they were leaving, but that someone would be back first thing in the morning. Apparently, I was not in concordance with this perceived abandonment. My brain wasn't able to process it properly, so I asked for the car keys. Without keys, you can't drive away. The request was politely declined, and the aforementioned plan was reiterated. From my hospital bed, all encumbered with wires and intravenous tubes, I repeated my demand for the keys with more assertiveness. I didn't want to be left alone, blind and broken, enveloped in the unfamiliar. My behest was again rejected, with kind and loving certainty. It had to be this way, but not for long, they told me, but apologetically, full of regret and torn by its reality. In a final plea for reconsideration, I looked at my father and spoke sternly. "Give me the fucking keys, dickweed!" He left the room more than a little taken aback by this aggressive outburst of his son. These were indeed uncharted waters for all and sundry. Someone told my family that I had no idea what I was saying that *head injuries are like that*. I can't imagine what everyone's faces were like after the verbal eruption, but, regardless, they had to leave.

It wouldn't be the only time I had an emotional intense reaction to a situation I failed to see the appeal of in those days. My mother would hear a nurse complaining about me. I had been rude and offended her while she was trying to do her job. She had wanted to take my temperature with an oral thermometer. I, conversely, did not want her to take my temperature with an oral thermometer, regardless of the act's banal and harmless nature. She cajoled me. She rationalized and reasoned with me. She was likely as personable and professional as could be expected on any day of a nurse's life. "Please," she said. "Just put this in your mouth for a minute."

"Why don't you stick it up your ass for a minute?" I retorted—not the response anyone in the medical community would like to hear from a fourteen-year-old, I suppose. I apparently didn't like her as much as the nurse whose smile I remember in the back of an ambulance. Needless to say, my mother wasn't pleased to hear anyone complain about her son as he was so nearly torn away in tragedy. My eyes had yet to even open, so outbursts were literally blindly targeted. Hell, she had gotten off easy compared to what I'd said to my old man. Besides, there were greater concerns than the unintended ululation of profanities barked by a teenager that still might die.

The only other story I recall hearing from those few days in Amherst not directly about my brain injury was when my sight came back. After some time in the hospital, under the watchful eyes of nurses, my head swelling had apparently gone down. When I awoke one morning, I was able to open my eyes just enough to see. I wanted a mirror. I would have obviously felt the swelling, the pain. My tongue likely probed the missing chunks in my teeth with disillusioned abandon. I can't be sure if I had any knowledge even then of my circumstances. Not fully. Could I recall the event itself? I have no idea. I could, however, see again, and I wanted a mirror to inspect what I could feel, to give visual shape and substance to something I knew was altered. Reluctantly, my mother gave into my insistence. A heartfelt expression of hope and reassurance undoubtedly chimed gently from her as she handed me the mirror. I looked at myself. "Leave me here to die alone. I'm too ugly to live."

She wept.

I can't relate too much about what they went through, my parents and siblings. It was never discussed in any great detail *after*. It was not likely a time anyone would want to recall in abundance. I do know of the uncertainty. The doctor in charge of monitoring me had a reputation for being less than thorough. Some folks might have even said he was objectively dismissive. All they knew was I had suffered a head injury and the doctor was waiting to see my progress. Inadequate attention was given, and answers were in short supply. In fact, he was going to simply send me home. I would go back to Pugwash, back into my parents' house and heal. Well, heal or die, I suppose. He could think of no further steps, apparently. As my parents are not neurologists, and nor was he, that was the plan. And it would have come to pass if it hadn't been for that nurse, the one whose smile I can still see in my mind twenty-eight years later. Upon hearing I was being released, she asked,

"So, the CT scan came back positive?".

"The *what*?" my mom inquired.

"They did send him to Moncton for a CT, right?'

"No, he hasn't been to Moncton," my parents responded.

"Do not let him go home until he gets to Moncton for a CT." It was more of a demand than a suggestion.

It was in the ambulance to Moncton that I saw that smile. She was leaning over me the whole way, smiling. The fluorescent lights of the ambulance were like a halo. She kept asking me to say her name, to keep me lucid. I remembered her name for over two decades. I wish I still could. I owe her my life.

In Moncton the CT scan revealed previously obscured and unknown facts. The full gravity of the situation became apparent. Not only had the membrane surrounding my brain been breached but my brain had suffered lacerations and contusions, what, years later, would be referred to as "significant damage" to my frontal lobe. In addition to this stark discovery was the presence of shards of skull fragments floating loose and uninhibited beneath. Had I been sent home I do not doubt I would have perished before too long.

It was in Moncton that my eyes opened completely. It was there, too, that my brain came to rest enough that I could retain information. I was still medicated—of this I am certain. I also had improved care based on the diagnosis gleaned from my CT. A charming student nurse from PEI was on hand often. She was only a few years older than me, less than a decade, and I felt a calmness around her. She was compassionate and had a vested interest in my well-being without seeming contrived or rehearsed. In general, the nurses there made me more comfortable with my situation, but the student nurse resonated with me a little more. Perhaps it was because the difference in years was that much less. Whatever the case, my overall experience was pleasant. I was able to begin to comprehend the seriousness of my situation; my perceptions were no longer shrouded in a density of chaos and numbness.

Sadly, more and more details have slipped away or became enmeshed in fantasy and false recollection over the years. The name of that student nurse from PEI was lost long ago, and her image in my mind is so vague as to inhibit the most generalized description. However, as I reflect on her, I assure you that the feeling of calm is recalled anew. There is a wonderful experience by and by, when you know that you are in the presence of a healer, someone who holds your health and well-being with utmost concern and respect. It's a situation I have been in repeatedly throughout my life. There have been doctors and nurses through the years that have struck a deep chord with me. It's like a reservoir of hope and faith in me and the benevolence that can reside in others. In Moncton I felt I was in good hands.

Being fourteen years old, I was to be housed in the children's ward of the hospital. I believe anyone under eighteen was relegated to the children's ward. This meant that for the three weeks or so that I was there, my roommates would change dramatically. On one of the two other beds could be a six-year-old or a sixteen-year-old, depending on the length of their stay. I was in for a long haul, as my injury was severe, and the prognosis required a delicate and methodical approach. The ward was divided into girls and boys, so naturally all my fellow guests were boys.

There was the young man on my left, a boy of eight or nine. He was to have his tonsils removed. His family was a constant presence. When the Nintendo the hospital had for the ward would come around and it was this kid's turn to play, he would often let his older brother play instead and just stare at the screen. When it was the younger brother's turn nothing else existed. He would not respond to his mother, the nurses, or anyone. After they took out his tonsils, he would wake the room (if not the whole hospital) with the kind of shrill, bone-piercing scream only a nine-year-old can make a 3 a.m. This would happen a couple times a night as the devoted and angelically patient nurse had to coax him into taking his medicine, in would seem the little scamp would find the process agonizing after surgery. One night the screams were interrupted and my muttering displeasure about it came to a halt. The fifteen-year-old across from me snapped, "Shut the fuck up!"

The fifteen-year-old and I talked a bit. The usual hospital thing started it off. That exchange of stories. The nuts and bolts of *what led you to be under the knife at a young age.* He had essentially disembowelled himself a smidge while trying to free up some brownie from a pan with an eight-inch kitchen knife. When they removed the bandages the first time to check the sutures, he didn't scream at a blood-curdling pitch but there was a notable volume to the bursts of profanity. There was anger in his undulations. It wasn't just anger at what was happening, the pain he was feeling—it was the anger of knowing that what was happening, the pain felt was the result of your actions. Your lack of forethought, perspective, or anticipation was the cause of your predicament. I could relate to an extent, but such things took longer to assimilate in my condition. I was unable to fully understand and absorb the full magnitude of my injury—in part because I had no memory of it. He, on the other hand, had the unadulterated footage to review. When the young man spoke of it, he seemed disappointed or even embarrassed, though he tried to laugh it off. This is a state of mind I would later come to know.

Due to the length of my stay, perhaps, I was granted few benefits. I got a little more time with the Nintendo a little more frequently. I can remember the taste and texture of that extra bowl of chocolate pudding I would get from time to time. One of the nurses used to joke kindly about my long hair spread out on my pillow as I slept through her nightly rounds. She would smile and suggest that, with hair so long, I should be called "Leanne," or something to that effect. I had my IV changed so many times I could practically do it myself—or so I thought. The same nurse chastised me when I did try to help by removing it myself, even though I had learned a decent amount from continuous observation. My veins tend to roll, so my introduction of any further complications was frowned upon. I received gifts and cards of well-wishing. News and messages were delivered from home via my family.

Then one day I was asked how much of my hair I wanted to keep. They needed to shave the front part of my head, but I could keep the length in the back, they said. Even though I was severely brain damaged, I had the sense not to opt for a mullet. I elected to have them shave my whole head; three years of growth and expression of individuality would be tied off, cut and bagged before my head was shaved clean for surgery. There may well still be a bag with that ponytail somewhere in my father's house. I was under, as they say, before the scissors and clippers were put to use. I closed my eyes on that gurney with tendrils of dark brown hair brushing my shoulders through the hospital gown as the anesthetic lulled me to sleep and I was rolled into the operating room for my surgery.

Dr. G performed the surgery, along with a plastic surgeon who would reconstruct with the assistance of a team of interns and nurses. I can't recall how long it took, only that it was significantly longer than expected. I can't imagine locating then extracting shards of my fractured skull was easy. My grandfather called from Ontario and found out first that I was out of surgery. He just happened to call as I was being wheeled out and the doctor was on his way to inform my parents. However, the fact my father found out from his father that I was out and not the doctor didn't sit well with him. He let the doctor know, with strong assertion, that it did not make a lot of goddamn sense that someone in Oshawa knew before he did that his son's operation was a success. That moment would pass. The important thing was that I was OK. My parents were given the ins-and-outs of the procedure.

I would be placed in intensive care. Where once I had hair, I was now decorated in a long scar. It starts beneath my right temple, just in front of my ear and travels up over the apex of my head behind the hairline to stop above my other temple. I got fifty-two staples, a number I'll never forget as I would count them later as they were being removed. I even held them in my hand. There was also medical-grade stainless steel mesh implanted. Two micro-thin layers were surgically installed to provide stability and support while the bone fused together, one inside my skull and one beneath the skin. The surgery was successful, but I was by no means in the clear.

I needed to be watched closely for several days after. Infection and rejection were very real concerns. Then, to make matters more sensitive to complication, a meningitis outbreak occurred in Moncton. Fresh out of brain surgery, I was high risk. Exposure and contraction would be a real fly in the ointment. The monitoring would now include my being tested for meningitis. It was precautionary on account of my not having been exposed and having been in as sterile an environment as one could be—but, nonetheless, the test had to be done post haste.

The test, from the patient's point of view, is a three-step process. First, curl up on your side in the fetal position, nice and tight. This stretches out your back and increases the softer tissue space between vertebrae. Then, once the doctor is satisfied you're in position and are not going to move, he takes a needle charged with a local anesthetic and pierces between vertebrae in your lower back. This freezes your spine so you cannot move or feel anything. Before the anesthetic kicks in, the pressure is surreal, as though there is simply no room for any more fluid in your spine. Just as it is at an almost unbearable level of discomfort, you go numb. You can hardly feel your legs as they are on the other side of the injection. The third phase is replacing the first needle with one that quietly takes in a supply of spinal fluid for testing. It essentially drips into the needle and collects. After enough fluid for testing has been procured, the needle is removed, and you lie there waiting for sensation to return. Not pleasant around the second step, but its brevity makes it tolerable. Of course, this is when all is going well.

I had the procedure done three times in three days. It was a safety precaution as I was fresh from under the knife and at high risk for infection. The first two times went as detailed above: first, get into a fetal position. Then endure a fierce and uncomfortable pressure before numbness sets in. Finish with a sample for the lab being drawn. The third and final time I had an extra experience at the end. It would seem that the spinal fluid wasn't dripping into the needle as freely as the previous two times. The doctor opted to remedy this by pulling back ever so slightly on the plunger of the needle lodged in my lower spine. I will remember the result for the rest of my life. A section of my spinal cord itself sucked to the side of the needle and my leg shot out, and a wave of agony passed quickly and with malevolence down my leg. It was like a single pulse of all the contusion, abrasion, burning, slicing, and shock you can fathom, a one-second broadcast of the purest agony careening down my rigid limb to vanish, leaving a wake of synaptic aftershock to echo a second later. To my valid yelp of pain, the doctor responded that it would be OK and "wouldn't happen again." No sooner did the last syllable pass his lips than my leg shot out stiff and anguished once more. If he did it again, I vowed I would deck him. It (thankfully) didn't happen again. Nor would there be need for further testing, as I was out of the danger zone of post-op. The experience left me with a bitter taste for the man and his nonchalance about my torment. It also gave me a litmus test of all sorts for pain. To this day I gauge all pain, every injury—no matter how potent, by those waves of agony.

The only other memory I have of my time in ICU is of a young man in the hospital bed to my left. He was perpendicular to me, and I had a clear view of him. His days-old scruff of a beard and his sweat-heavy locks were drenched auburn. The tubes and wires, the beeps and chimes of monitors all remain unembellished by descriptives.

I watched daily as his family and nurses came to his bedside. His head would roll this way and that in response to familiar voices, as his eyes would roll into his head, fleeing those damn fluorescent lights. I remember the devotion and strength of his mother as she fed him as she once did in his infancy, when he was helpless and dependent. I remember him. I will never forget. His name is lost to my travels, but those images will never leave me. The level of his trauma, the severity of it, were surreal to me. I didn't yet know what had happened. All I could perceive was like a somnambulist desperation to awaken from the bad dream. I perceived a desire for him to awaken from the state he was in, to escape back to bygone days. They all wanted it—his family and the doctors, they wanted it. I could feel it. He wanted it. I could feel he did. We all could. No one could tell if it was even within reach, but the abundance of love held doubt at considerable distance. I felt that too.

I didn't know the details about him. Having had my own wild ride through the hospitalized rigmarole, I was not fully able to process what I was seeing. I could easily recognize and relate to the cavalcade of white coats and scrubs, family and staff. I could see and acknowledge the devastating condition the young man was in. I could tell he was older than me. I could tell that his situation was far more dire than mine. I could not, however, relate any of it to my own situation. His story was clearly different. It was tragic and excruciating, but not my own. My young age, the post-op meds, and my newly acquired brain injury impeded my need to know, to understand what had happened. How was it that a sixteen-year-old boy was reduced to a level of need he had not known in fifteen years? The notion terrified me.

In under a week, I was moved from ICU back the Children's Ward. The threat of meningitis had abated, and I was to remain a week in the ward under watchful eyes as I healed from a successful surgery. The nurse from PEI had returned home to finish her studies and no one would be screaming from the loss of tonsils. I relaxed as I knew extra pudding and Nintendo privileges would return forthwith. I had a feeling that all was and would be just fine as the orderlies and nurses transferred me to my bed and left.

The guy across from me was about sixteen. He was a hockey player who'd lost the "ball" of his elbow. He said it had broken off during a particularly destructive check. He also asked if I had just come from ICU. Just like that.

"Did you just come from ICU?" he asked.

"Yes. . ."

"Was there a guy there all fucked up, like with tubes and stuff?"

I admit I was taken off guard when he asked. It was a blunt question, but I could tell he was compelled by a need only the heart could muster. He knew him, you see. They had played hockey together back in the day. He admitted that they had grown apart over the years, but he knew him and his family. He also knew what had happened to him. I listened with curiosity, compassion, and keen interest as he told me what had occurred.

Out at the lake one day, not long before, the young man in ICU had opted to ignore his friend's advice and dive into the refreshing waters to escape the heat of late summer in New Brunswick. He'd opted to dive where they'd advised not to. As I listened intently, the guy across from me explained that he wasn't there but had heard that the water was too shallow. He told me that after diving into the lake, ten feet below the surface, the young man crashed headfirst into the rocky bottom. He'd suffered massive head trauma and broken his neck in a lake not far from the hospital.

"He was a really good hockey player. And now he has to learn to do everything again. Talk. Walk. Shit. He'll probably never fuck again."

I heard all this before the guy across from me knew my story. I never told him. It seemed wrong somehow, so I kept it to myself. How could I speak with the truth of my experience dawning on me, the whole truth? Until that point I had yet to absorb the stark reality, the indisputable fact that I could have died, or at best that I too could have found myself in perpetual need of assistance. I felt lucky. I felt frightened. I felt entirely overwhelmed by the magnitude of possibilities. For the first time I was in awe of how much worse it could have been. It was both humbling and empowering. There must have been a reason I'd fared so much better.

I would like to believe that these words were the beginning of my discernment of an answer.

2

HIGH SCHOOL: THE UNDEFINED STRUGGLE

A month of hospitalization is marked now, nearly thirty years later, by darkness. The majority of those days are lost—buried and forgotten. My recollection has been consumed by the unyielding fires of active trauma. My brain, in tatters, was unable to grasp the details of its predicament. Most of my memory of that time is constructed from anecdotal, third-person accounts of the events that had come to pass. Further askew by time's distortions and personal misconception, I can only relay history in fragments.

This much is certain. I left the hospital in Moncton to return home to Nova Scotia. Pugwash has a facility for adults for those with special needs on account of mental and developmental issues. That, however, was not my destination. Though the Sunset Community Adult Rehabilitation Centre had existed in my hometown for nearly a century, I was not destined to become a resident. I was to return home. I was to return to junior high. After all, the operation had been a success. I was patched up and cosmetically fit, prime to return to normal life as a fourteen-year-old boy of the early nineties in rural Nova Scotia.

I was still not yet cognizant enough to be aware of the reactions around me, to be able to register and process the reluctant compulsion of friends and classmates as they hesitantly approached me to gander and inquire. My shorn head and pronounced scar were a stark contrast to their memories of me, as were my timid demeanour and languid responses. Some wept, some stared in silence. My friends clamoured to offer aid and support. It all washed over me, still in a neurological stasis of disbelief about what had occurred. Even the two young asshole hicks that mocked me daily didn't register at first. There was just too much going on all at once, all the time.

Something atavistic was occurring behind my eyes, between frontal and apex, my brain was flicking switches on or off as the situation required. By times, I absorbed all the stimuli as best I could or limited it to a minimum intake lest unpredictable responses manifested. Neither empowering nor subduing, my mental state was precariously balanced in a stupor of numb acceptance. Teachers and students alike gave me a berth—not of understanding, but of curiosity, wonder, and sympathy—those two assholes excluded, of course.

When I couldn't remember a time, an adventure we had shared, my friends would provide more detail, trying to trigger a memory. When I would stare blankly at nothing in particular during class, the teacher would just continue. My emotional mind would acknowledge these moments, even when my conscious mind fell short. I could feel the desire to get through, the yearning for a former self that I could not recognize let alone provide. Empathy, a fledgling trait, would whisper through the din or silence, assuring me that I could ease their concerns.

I just had to try really fucking hard.

It was early in these days that I began to experience the active effects of memory loss. I felt the absence of joy and a twinge of sadness when friends would respond with knee-jerk reactions of disbelief that I couldn't recall this or that as they offered more detail in hopes of spawning a vague recollection in me of days past. It was and remains disheartening how one must reconstruct a lost memory, more so when it cannot be accomplished. I had lost even the idea that memories were missing and to this day still have expansive lacunas. This from a brain that was once near photogenic. My dismay was displayed in nonchalant expressions on the faces of those that knew and loved me.

Yet still I had no recollection of what I had lost, just the newly acquired knowledge that it was not to be found.

Obviously, I had to try really fucking hard. There is no documentation to refer to, no clinical record of my state. I was in recovery without the knowledge that I was. Not only was there no external acknowledgement of possible ramifications and real-life consequences, but my ability to decipher the array of information was severely impeded. I felt displaced into the familiar. Simultaneously, I was thrust into undefined struggles. All I knew before about myself and my life, was to be reacquainted with, remembered, or relearned.

There were frequent reminders and assurances that I had once been brilliant. It was constantly affirmed to me that I was smart and capable, with other people's memories of me reflecting the unspoken recognition and subsequent desire for a return of the Lenny Roach they knew. Their encouragement was a catalyst of sorts, I suppose. At bare minimum it was a better alternative to the ignorant and disparaging remarks of those two ignorant young men who'd mocked me. That negative influence notwithstanding, the empathetic and heartfelt words of encouragement compelled me. I wanted to be, if anyone, the young man they described.

Something of my former self still did reside within the enveloping uncertainty that waned and advanced, ebbed and flowed indiscriminately in concurrence with an esoteric biorhythm I am trying to comprehend even now. I needed to believe in something, as so much was missing or undefined. I needed to believe that the young man in the mirror and the young man they described were one and the same, or at least be able to merge into a singularity from which a perceivable universe could emerge, given a certain slant of insight.

I was basically never given any limitations beyond the words of those two insensitive jerks who hadn't enough knowledge between them to do more than repeat the same nonsense about learning to fly. Whether it was a lack of understanding or acceptance of the new conditions, or the desire for a predetermined normalcy, all involved within the inner circle of recuperation would proceed as though nothing had changed beyond the obvious. We were plausibly denying some aspects due to lack of information. Uninformed and unprepared, I commenced an unguided journey through a labyrinth of cerebral reconstitution.

I must admit I cannot be sure of any of our responses, or our behaviour as a whole or individually—not in the beginning, anyway, those days lost to nothing more than the passage of time. Perhaps some can remember in their forties the surreal plethora of experience that was the cyclone of hormones and discovery relegated to a fourteen-year-old human embedded indiscriminately into life, but I struggle fruitlessly to recall much. I can only assume there were various trials and tribulations for me, as there was for anyone. I can only similarly assume I had a harder time, as I still do. Those bleak and frightening memories of a silent, darkened bedroom wherein I would interrogate my mind into fits of desperate outbursts. I remember the frustration I felt when I couldn't overcome the confusion, when I struggled and strained to retain new information. Those uncharted waters still lap the shores of my self-actualization.

I would make my way through the halls, going from one classroom to the next, with a passive detachment. Somewhat removed from where I was and where I was heading, I would trudge forward, loosely engaged in idle chatter or lost in abstract thought devoid of fundamentally cohesive context. The hair I had started to grow out as an initiate metalhead back in the sixth grade having been shaved and discarded in preparation for surgery a month earlier, I wore a Metallica "Kill 'Em All" trucker cap constantly. The cap was to conceal the budding stubble and obscure the scar that arched just behind my hairline, from temple to temple.

I was given upon request exemption from the traditionally upheld dictum of no hats in school as not only did I advantageously admit to feeling self-conscious about my appearance but because that same appearance was deemed a potential distraction to fellow students. An easy case for both explanations was plausible as the bilateral scarring gave the impression of the stitching one would see on a baseball. It was hard not to stare, I would assume, primarily because the bathroom mirror at home enticed me to do just that. Why should anyone else respond differently?

The moodiness, the awkwardness, and the overall behavioural shifts were common hallmarks of any young man of that age when hormones and sense of self take on more integral roles in everyday life. Though perhaps the potency of mine was by times more pronounced, it would have been easy to dismiss my altered state as nothing more than teenage angst. After all, weren't most of my classmates and friends undergoing similar undulations of temperament and decorum? It is human nature to seek a definition for any situation that is undesirable as temporary, a phase that will pass; likely, it was the same with me.

Whether it was a result of the trauma, the naturally occurring flood of hormonal contradictions or a combination of both, I can only assume that the hopes of those within my inner circle of friends and family was that my situation would improve over time, that I would resume the life I'd lived before as a sensitive and intelligent young man with potential in some notable abundance. I, too, hoped for such an outcome and believed it was possible. Like so much belief, it's often built on the disbelief of the alternative. I had no reason to accept it couldn't be possible as no contradictory voice was to be heard, no prognosis had been offered to disavow the notion that I was going to be OK. It would just take a lot of work.

So, I set about doing the work—the same work I had intended to take up before the fall, before the surgery, before the myriad new challenges that would assail me throughout my recovery. Classroom life had been of only passing interest to me even before, depending on the subject and level of interest injected by the teacher. Knowledge and learning were, however, of interest. I enjoyed learning new things; information granted me insight, spurred my imagination, and fueled my curious nature. My intent was to continue to approach my studies with the same varying degree of interest. I had always been able to retain information, whether or not I was invested, at least enough to pass the tests and exams as needed. If the subject matter interested me or was presented in a way that grabbed my attention, I would excel a little more. Going forward, I believed that this would again be the case and at first it appeared to be so. Of course, a little slack was extended as I had just returned from the hospital and was a full month behind, an arrangement that was beneficial though ultimately misleading. It would not be long before struggles and challenges would crop up around me. Forgetfulness, distraction, and disconnection would bear forth the fruit of frustration. The remainder of my junior high years would be an under-the-wire slide from semester to semester. The course load was predetermined by the curriculum, and I had no option but to acquiesce to the mandate, whether or not I was interested. It wouldn't be until senior high, Grades 10 through 12, that I could select classes that interested me, classes I believed could keep my mind focused and not merely faltering about in lethargic distraction.

A major factor in the courses I would choose was not the subject matter itself, or even the proverbial doors they would potentially open in the future. It was the quantity and quality of the students with whom I would be spending my time that most influenced my choices. There were essentially three levels of academia at Pugwash District High School: university prep, advanced, and a more generalized or remedial level. I opted for the former as the latter two tiers were characterized by larger number of students with varying levels of intellectual discipline. More people meant more voices, more distractions, and more sensory intake that my brain would need to ignore or balance. The university prep classes were small, often under a dozen students per class. Furthermore, I was well acquainted with most of the students enrolled in them—most of the young men and women in my English class, for example, had gone to kindergarten with me. Some of the students in the class were friends from pre-teenager days of summer bikes and winter toboggans. I was comforted by the familiarity as I struggled with strange new obstacles. They, too, were familiar with me, both before and after my accident. They knew me to be intelligent and unusual, creative and funny. They knew I had suffered trauma and were supportive and empathetic, often offering assistance when I was clearly struggling to grasp a concept or solve a problem.

Though I was not often able to achieve the scholastic quota that was the objective of the course load for which we all had opted, I was never criticized or discouraged for these shortcomings. For three years it would be the same classmates, friends by the end if not before, striving in our own ways to achieve, to accomplish the goal of something better in the future.

It would take twenty-five years before I would understand that my taking those challenging classes was integral to my recuperation. I was pushing my damaged and uncertain brain to its utter limits as I stumbled through chemistry, biology, and physics at a level meant for those with lofty aspirations of scholarships and letters affixed to their names. It was a three-year boot camp of mental exercises and rehabilitation. For the most part, my marks were shit, but my condition did bring a unique perspective. So much of the world was almost like new to me that I would make a child's inquiry with adult insight, a deeper reflection on the basest of facts. This was in part due to my still wandering mind, but any and all answers I could get were somehow necessary (Being lost and free are not that different I suppose).

I may not have been able to achieve the A's or B's that had once come so easily. Frustration may have driven me to punch holes in the walls of my bedroom or tear out my own hair in the dark silence of the night. Confusion and disbelief were still stalking me like the shadowed memory of my former self.

Tormented, I pushed onward. Not always giving my all, but always *being* my all. I would continue to take the classes that challenged, that demanded more of me. Though I wasn't as successful as I would have been had I not fractured my skull and lacerated my frontal lobe, I refused to relegate myself to a path more easily traversed. I believe it was the subconscious rewards of improved deduction and speculation that spurred me on. My memory was improving, and old memories were flocking back to roost as they once did. I was unable to excel in any one subject but again could retain a myriad of intellectual tidbits. Random facts would anchor themselves to the soft tissue before my mind's eye, facilitating quick access. I would help take the PDHS "Reach for the Top" team to the provincial trivia championship one year on account of a newly blossoming orchard of miscellaneous knowledge.

The orchard bore fruit of hope.

Honestly, I had to attend high school an extra year. I didn't have enough credits to graduate with the same friends with whom I had spent all those hours over all those years. The effects of the two months of evoked chaos from the second semester of Grade 11 echoed through the halls into the final days of my return to Grade 12.

One day the echoes were interrupted by a request over the PA for a friend and me to report to the vice-principal's office. The year near completion, I cringed at the possibilities. The vice-principal was also the guidance counsellor, so the reasons for our being beckoned were potentially numerous. When we met in the second-floor hallway after leaving our respective classes, we discussed the possible reason for the summons. My friend and I agreed that a very plausible reason was us peddling hash on school property.

After synching our story entirely on plausible deniability, we walked toward the office knowing that if we saw the boys in blue, we would be irrevocably fucked.

We were wrong. We had been pulled out of class to discuss the remarkable scores we'd achieved on the standardized aptitude tests. We were consistently in the high nineties. Apparently, this could open doors to any university in the country, a point she punctuated by sliding brochures across the desk that we did not hesitate to ignore.

In hindsight, it was an affirmation that I had made great progress. Perhaps opportunity that I missed was simply acknowledging the validity of that accomplishment.

3
I CAN SEE IT COMING FROM A MILE AWAY

There are undeniable extremes that come with brain damage.

Beyond the nature of the injury itself (how it occurred and the extent of the damage), there are extremes in how the brain responds. There are sudden shifts from subjective normalcy into the objectively abnormality. These shifts result in a variety of changes, both perceivable and not, that are beyond control. Mood swings and emotional instability become hard-wired into the psyche, and one finds themselves at their mercy.

I am unable to ignore or silence numerous internal phantasms that only speak of ill-tidings and misgivings. The creation of hypothetical problems that demand immediate responses are troubling waters to navigate. Frustration raging in my mind as it grasps wildly at the past, pulling negative memory out of forgotten darkness to again ruminate upon. All that has happened is again scrutinized. Imagine if all that you've suffered, all that you lost wass lit by a seething anger. The life you could have had has been ripped from you unceremoniously and you are right to be angry.

Aspirations have been replaced by challenges.

When that frustration took on a particular flavour, I opted for distraction, thinking as little as I could as each thought was a potential misstep into different tribulations. I channelled the energy into my work, my art, avoiding others as best I could, as I was known to be unbearable while navigating such tributaries. Primarily, I prepared for things to get brackish. The deep anger that flails and rages would churn up all the silt in my mind. It muddied the water with thoughts of failure, loss, weakness, and dread. Soon no light would be visible, clouded and stifled by the detritus of days past. The choices I'd made and the regrets they carried set adrift before my mind's eye like photographs in flood waters. I knew what came next. I could see the churning in the distance, feel the current shifting. There was no fighting the impending undertow. Soon I would be pulled under again and I no longer fought it.

In the beginning I would struggle, try to break the surface or find some degree of footing in the murky depths. Now I just took a deep breath and sank passively into the dark, seeking neither rescue nor reprieve.

When all I heard was whispers of defeat and all I saw was futility it was best that I removed myself from the world. It was preferable that I suffered alone, as I was not able to detail what ailed me. It was better that I distanced myself, isolating in darkness and introspection. The ideal situation is having time and space to prepare. I had become familiar with the warning signs. A desperate resignation followed on the heels of unwarranted and directionless outbursts. Futility and disenchantment in the wake of frustration, I succumbed fully to an inner monologue of self-loathing. Distance of time and space became beyond necessary. Abject irritability being condition enough to spare friends and family from the displeasure of trying to navigate my moods and outburst I would hide myself away. The latter condition of depression and defeat is worse. The frustration I can at least explain, rationally or otherwise. It's when I become fully crestfallen that I find myself at a great disadvantage. The very idea of trying to express myself seemed such a fruitless endeavour as to not warrant an effort; I settled for cynicism and silence. No one needed to see that.

A quiet wall of negativity developed between me and the world; I was prone to lashing out at those that intrude upon my misery. Whether I am being dismissive or callous, I am known to respond to things that are kind and nurturing with disapproval. Propping myself up before caring eyes and clearly in distress, I would practically invite whomsoever closer before lashing out. More often than not this would result in regret and discomfort later. So now, when I feel that nihilistic demon beginning to stir in the cerebral shadows, I retreat into solitude, unwilling to allow a modicum of its noxious words to breathe toxicity in the air between myself and another. There is no good anyone can do for me, and I will characteristically only create disharmony.

In my teens this retreat into darkness and reclusive disenchantment would mean days of unlit hours behind my bedroom door, refusing contact of any kind, pulling out my hair and throwing cherished things about in the dark. It was as though I could feel my brain trying to arrange the pieces of the day or week into something it could decipher. Thoughts succeeded in superimposing themselves in unrelenting succession. I longed for a moment of reprieve. My brain would ache and labour to catalogue events and feelings that had transpired throughout just a single day of high school. Exhausted and overwhelmed, I would eventually collapse into slumber with an empty stomach and a head that throbbed incessantly. There was little doubt this behaviour was cause for concern. I am also certain that I would have greeted that concern with disinterest at best as I was already in the depths of post-traumatic repercussions and incapable of absorbing any more external stimuli, no matter their source.

These days I do essentially the same thing. I close the door and kill the lights. Not as much gets thrown around or destroyed as it used to because I have learned to suppress the urge years ago. I still keep tight lips as to why I seclude myself. I usually just tell people I'm sleeping. I frequently boast about my ability to sleep for up to sixteen hours at a time—it's a ruse many likely see through, but it is accepted as a reasonable response and further questions are rarely forthcoming after that explanation. It is, for the most part, true by the way. A high percentage of those hours I spent in dark and quiet bedrooms were indeed spent asleep. It was never a deep slumber, and I awoke sporadically. Ushered to consciousness by shards of thoughts that only seemed to exist between sleep and the waking life, I'd stare into the darkness and contemplate that sudden shard of thought that had wedged itself into my mind.

Eventually, and in unmeasured intervals, I would drift into deep sleep where my weary brain could rest and recuperate. Dreaming and neurological maintenance being integral, though the former is not often remembered, I allowed my body to do the behind-the-scenes work that I never question. Let the amygdala ignite into a flurry of increased activity, the purpose of which remained elusive. I would allow the limbic system to do a house-cleaning of the garbled and frivolous, clearing away the clutter in hopes of facilitating new focus, new perspectives.

During those hours I may have come in and out of sleep a dozen times to weep or shudder, cringe or seethe. From beneath the covers, I may have muttered to myself about all that hurt me, all my fears and anxiety. A stream of unrestrained thoughts may have poured into the darkness, muffled by pillows and solitude, heard by none but me. I may have cursed my choices, my situation, my life itself in a cathartic diatribe. Enveloped in an isolation with which I had become all too familiar, I no longer resisted and began letting the demon speak, giving him his time in court to plead the case for the futility of all I knew and all I was. Simultaneously, I gave myself time to deliberate and postulate. There could be no escape, so I surrendered willingly to the turmoil of depressed and dismal thoughts.

Len Roach

So often have I endured hours of self-inflicted torment that I knew I would survive as I had before.

There may be neither conquering nor vanquishing of that dreadful, dark spectre in my mind, but there is also no defeat. Every time, I eventually emerge from the quiet cover of self-imposed confinement. Every time, I am better than before I went in. Sweating out the toxins and purging me of poisons is not a ritual I seek willingly, but I can see its necessity from a mile away. I can sense the impending moments of sorrowful introspection as they approach and can ready myself for their arrival. I'd equate this to seeing a horizon cloaked in storm grey, dreary shades progressively saturating the sky. As the clouds get closer, enveloping the world in a lachrymose shroud, I know I will soon be staring through a windowpane streaked with rivulets; my reflection in the glass, faint and scarcely recognizable, will render me transfixed and vulnerable as I wait for the storm to pass.

4
Perpetuating Repercussive Cycles

Just behind my eyes, faulty and distinctive, is my orbitofrontal cortex, a convergence of neurons where cognizance and consequence meet with a frequency measured in milliseconds. It's a summit of impulses, reactions, perceptions, and judgements that precedes and succeeds every choice, every decision.

Language and motor skills are dependent on the stability of the OFC, as are various high faculties. Rats with scientifically strategic lesions were known to have a penchant for instantaneous gratification, their rational brain hindered from influencing the flights of fancy their emotional brains proposed. Long-term goals are exchanged for short-term pleasure, synthetic or otherwise. Options are weighed without the consideration of outcomes. As it was for rats in cages, it has been for me.

My first severe brain injury would leave scarring and dead tissue. When the bone that creates the orbital part of my skull above my right eye shattered, shards lacerated the folds, creating cerebral lesions. My inability to properly access and use available information was the outcome. It was not a permanent state of being and the frequency of the condition has lessened through the years. Nonetheless, there has been a plethora of occasions in the past three decades wherein I've found myself at a great disadvantage as it pertained to making beneficial decisions.

Anyone who has had the experience of waking up hungover and wallowing in disbelief of their actions from the night before is familiar with the effects of alcohol on the prefrontal cortex.

Risk assessment and inhibition having been drowned out and washed away by an excess of libations that only seemed to reinforce their own propagation, one is dumbfounded by the results of actions determined obviously detrimental in hindsight. The steady release of neurotransmitters serotonin, dopamine, and endorphins keep an inebriated brain gleefully making spontaneous decisions repeatedly as the ability to gauge plausible repercussions drifts ever farther away. Brief and frivolous rewards become enticing. Intoxicated, the cerebral acuity needed to perceive the dire truths of the situation is effectively stifled, if not silenced. So, the risks are increasingly less perilous and the choices are more flippant. The congestion of the mesolimbic pathway remains, risk and reward press bumper to bumper, until the drink runs dry, and one awakens in a fog of confusion and regret.

On account of the damage that I had suffered at fourteen, I was familiar with this kind of situation without the amplification begotten of the drink. I would respond instantly and excessively to situations. The effects of such emotional outburst were seldom, if ever, as devastating or lasting as when I would make decisions disregarding the truth of my situation. Cognizant only of the immediate, I was not unwilling but unable to consider any possible future. The possible outcomes, positive or negative, were simply not derived from relative and influential memory as they were not in the moment available for counsel, having been misplaced in my travels. Minutes, hours, or even days later, I would eventually have the flood of plausible consequences assail me. Anxiety and panic, depression and desperation would all rally for dominance of the consequential new state of affairs.

Whether it meant unemployment (it often did) or that I was again single (it often did), I would be left bewildered and taken aback by my lack of forethought.

Trying simultaneously to piece together the events that led me to make such a snap decision, I would find myself forced to rely on the very faculties that had failed me. The valuation of potential risks associated with the consequences and theoretical behavioural flexibility required to navigate them represent myriad possibilities. I was frequently in a far more precarious situation than I had been prior. My faith and confidence in my deductive and executive functions shaken by my reckless indulgence, I would seek instantaneous gratification. Impulsivity would don a different hat and I would turn to the drink. Like putting gasoline on a grease fire, things would not improve.

When I was drinking or on coke, my ability to perceive consequence was practically abolished by the need for instant thrills. At my worst, the thoughts and feelings of friends and family were inconvenient to acknowledge as I clambered from mistake to mistake, lapse to lapse. During the most destructive times of substance abuse, I was nearly sociopathic in my lack of regard for others and often oblivious to the future that waited beyond egocentric caprice. Tomorrow didn't matter and next week didn't exist. When I was a drunk and fiend, I knew only the cycle of stimulus and shame that enveloped me and determined my every choice. My prefrontal cortex, already scarred and fragile, was stupefied by deluges of booze and drugs. Disinhibited, I found impulsivity led me from plateaus of moral and ethical considerations into the mire of superficial, libertine avarice.

I had always had trouble weighing pros and cons until I stopped weighing them all together. I was never certain of any choice I made—those of the life-altering variety, anyway. The passage of time to me was somewhat askew, so making long-term plans was alien to me. An integral aspect of the impulsivity and all subsequential matters was an inability to envision a future at all. To attempt to visualize a future would require the acknowledgment of my mistakes and bad decisions or at best invite such an overwhelming barrage of possibilities that I would be nearly catatonic with indecision. That level of stress and shame was not appealing, so I would embrace the frivolity of the instant reward. Spontaneously, I would quit a job or cause a breakup. Drama in my wake, I would stride recklessly into psychosis and things deplorable.

It doesn't serve to detail the pain I bestowed on those around me. The chaos and audaciousness witnessed having affected so many in diverse ways, I simply do not have the insight to do it justice. I can just be aware that my inability to acknowledge clear evidence of the ill-advised had become insufferable to everyone, including me.

The trauma of brain damage having never been explored or explained by any semblance of a specialised follow up, I was left to struggle with associated issues without guidance or understanding. The temptations of youth were difficult to ignore and equally difficult to refuse. My memory of the past was partial and vague, so I lacked the reference points and influence. As any given day felt in many ways akin to a new beginning, the previous day was essentially forgotten or at least ignored. I could not seem to hold any contemplative inclination for very long. Fragments of memory would disrupt incomplete thoughts, disabling cohesive decision-making. When presented with any choice I would often adopt indifference as my demeanour.

The question of "Why not?" was one I was unable to answer succinctly. It became an default, flashcard excuse for whatever action I would take. It was this defect in cognitive thought that factored into substance abuse. The escape from confusion, frustration, and lament I knew as a result of my injury were easily and instantly sidestepped with booze and drugs.

LSD and mushrooms were a means to strip away some of a reality that was overbearing; any lasting effects weren't worth thinking about. Mushrooms being seasonal and acid scarce, my drug of choice was cannabis. I am adamant that no lasting ill effects from cannabis remain, directly or indirectly. Even during those slow-moving days of my youth in rural Nova Scotia as a teenager, the worst I can say of pot is that it made me lazy and distracted. The impulse to smoke it whenever and wherever possible only hindered me in ways I considered superficial.

Too stoned to go to the dojo, too stoned to go home in time for supper, too stoned to study. Whatever it was couldn't be that important. Besides, there would always be other meals, other tests, and other opportunities for whatever I had opted not to do.

The THC and the CBD calmed me and helped streamline the matrix of random thoughts and feelings that would too often assail me. That instant relief from a brain prone to misfires and synaptic blizzards was much desired if not essential. Had it remained merely marijuana with occasional acid trips or shroom journeys I would likely have had an easier time. However, by the time I had reached grade eleven I was an unapologetic drug fiend, willing and wanting of anything I could get my hands on, illicit or prescribed. A few Percodan one recess in the cafeteria, taken without hesitation or reflection, would lead to weeks of numbness. I have only sparse memories of my time as a pharmaceutical zombie marauding about my life—and all of them are disturbing. A direct result of an impulsive choice to guinea pig myself with, at the time, unidentified pills pilfered from a medicine cabinet was a nearly two-month addiction that rendered me emaciated and deranged.

"I wonder what they do?" a friend asked.

"I'll find out," I replied on a whim, washing them down with a Sprite. I awoke the next morning with no memory of what followed. Reality vanquished, I wanted more until the supply was depleted.

The malfunctions of impulse control would have been more manageable had alcohol not eventually taken the reins, exasperating my condition. My nineteenth birthday meant I could legally drink pretty much anywhere at any time. It would ultimately become my addict's impulse when life would throw me the unexpected. Might as well have a drink, right? Fired from a job? Drink. Girl ended things? Drink. Did someone die? Drink. Is it another boring Tuesday? Might as well drink.

Whenever events would leave me brooding and wallowing, the drink was there to numb my soul and subdue my brain. The fact that it lowered inhibitions and clouded judgement was neither here nor there. In light of whatever torment or sorrow that had put the drink in my hand, the consequences of getting shitface-hammered were irrelevant. Though this temporary indifference would often lead to further calamity, my damaged and intoxicated brain had no interest in, or faculty for, deterring me from destructive spontaneity. Likewise, it had little concern for those affected. Often, my primary concern was getting the stimulants I needed to keep me drinking. Forethought wasn't much more than a dismissive acknowledgment that if I passed out I would potentially awaken to sobering truths. With no pride whatsoever I admit to very derelict periods of my life where alcohol and cocaine transmuted me into a base and dastardly version of myself. Impulsivity having opened the door to spurious satisfaction, I was no longer able to discern an alternative. I lived for the instantaneous supplemental and it, in return, numbed me to the torment of it's repercussions. Broken tools cannot be repaired. Feed the demons so they may still whisper lies over a truth that was ever more evident.

Normal coping methods were foreign to me, always had been. Damage to my orbitofrontal cortex had made my limbic system faulty and unreliable. Where some would have a multitude of memories from which to build a template of rational decisions, I had an inkling of an idea that was blackened and redacted by scars and shadows. The need for serenity at any cost superseded the need for consistency or reason. Without knowledge of impairment, how the fuck was I supposed to adjust to accommodate for neurological shortcomings? Impulsivity brought instantaneous gratification and consequences I was unable to envision for lack of a comparative recollection. A daisy chain of regretful choices that spanned decades may have been avoided had I known the extent of the encephalopathy, had someone bothered to inform me.

5
"ARE YOU OK?"

Often throughout my culinary career I have had that feeling of eyes on me, the stillness of uncertainty as coworkers seemed to be stepping lightly around me. Some aspect of my intensity or whatnot would fluster the air around me in such a way, unperceived by me, that someone would ask "Are you OK?"

Normally I was, just focused. After so many years of persistence and laborious devotion in professional kitchens, it would be reasonable to assume I was just a burnt-out curmudgeon. In a lot of ways, I am. I am not the only one. There is a significant number of tired old chefs and cooks still grinding away, often for lack of anything else to do. I have those moments, but it wasn't always the case. In the early years I would still look stern and unimpressed as I rocked the dish pit or prepped *garde manger*. Later, as a sous chef, my demeanour invoked feelings of concern from those on my brigade.

Obviously, there would be times that my air of intensity was in fact borne of legitimate frustration, like plans going askew as the result of miscalculation or the unforeseen. Everyday life would, of course, chime in with some new fuckery to impede or distract. Generally speaking, I was just focusing intently. It was and is necessary for me. When tasks are delicate or time-sensitive and I have a vested personal interest, I have no option but to channel everything to them. Every micro-burst of synaptic impulse must be in the name of it, all under the umbrella named cuisine, in this case. I used to know, but recently forgot, the Japanese word for such devoted and serious focus, having learned it when a colleague asked me, her sous chef, "Are you OK?" The word and definition I learned from my Japanese cook was perfect. I found comfort in that word and the notion that there was a name for my frame of mind in any language.

It wasn't just in kitchens that I employed this focus. It had become instinctual, an acquired and required practice created from necessity and honed to satisfaction from high school on. My brain would leap on endless, boundless tangents if I didn't willfully enforce direction and attention. I'd go as far as obedience, in the early days of TBI life. At times, a near exhausting strain, a desperate pulling of the reins with Aesop undertones, would eclipse the world around me. Trying to achieve a glimmer of the light that shone when it was so easy, I had to fight through doubt and exasperation with every challenge. Give me dopamine. Give me sweet serotonin. Give me success in this task. There could be no distraction.

My eyes set hard under a furrowed brow of intent as I would devote my attention to my labours. From description I gather it is a resting face of formidable seriousness. I am unaware of either my surroundings or my expression as I stomp about, all the while muttering to myself in stern baritone. All consciousness gravitates to the task at hand and the tasks to come. The term herding cats comes to mind when I think of the bad days early on. I kept at it though, kept setting my eyes on the action I was performing while simultaneously giving my brain a reprieve from its delinquent wanderings, girdling all the neuropathic energy toward achieving my desired results. I would muster up stability to the best of my ability. Notwithstanding is the degree of success. It was an unsatisfactory win-loss record at first. I had to keep fighting though. I had to keep trying to train my brain again to observe, analyze, and retain. I had to teach it that cerebral juggling act of multitasking. Life as a cook proved to be a gymnasium of Herculean affect.

Over the years, as I climbed the ranks of a professional kitchen brigade, the mental tools and tendencies I acquired and developed on my post-trauma travels through teenage years not only served me advantageously but improved to the point that myriad events could be occurring in ruthless succession under my guidance without incident. I was able to not only conduct and orchestrate my own interactions and responses, but guide the success of others. I could call the line, assign and assess duties, and maintain a catalogue of data pertaining to guests, chits, inventory, and the timing in between all pertinent matters. Prep lists and orders, staff and purveyors all remained within reach of comprehension. The slow build of responsibility that comes with the professional kitchen paired nicely with my need for expression and desire to feast gluttonously on the hormonal rewards of success, the scrumptious flavour of endorphins and the delicacy of serotonin. Right-brain gratified by knowledge and left-brain gleeful for creation and expression made for a rewarding experience across those respective hemispheres. The balance played exquisite melodies with neuropsychological instruments as I would chore away passionately and enthusiastically, my face devotionally stern.

6
"Where's My Hair?"

I woke up in bed. Not unusual or unexpected as I would more than often wake up in bed, the events of the night before notwithstanding.

À propos, my back was arching slightly in response to the unfamiliar feel of the flaccid mattress beneath a weary body. My hand instinctively sought to run fingers through shoulder-length hair as they led my arms skyward in the rejuvenating exercise of ritualistic awakening.

"Where's my hair?"

It was my first and only thought. Perhaps I mouthed the words inaudibly, perhaps not. In my head, the question sounded off loud and insistent, breaking a silence both familiar and undefined. Akin to the post-naissance wail of life, the words heralding that something had gone askew revived me to a more astute consciousness.

Something was different. Something had changed.

The first taste of a new reality had yet to be poured fully and my palate screamed in confusion as to the tannin and viscosity. The immediate dilemma was embodied fully in the first thought. A vain question with menacing undertones broke the silence.

"Where's my hair?"

The question, an inquisitive evocation beckoning me to waking life, was followed by other phrases that were less personal but far more practical. The succession goes as follows: the first three thoughts when I awoke in the Foothills Medical Centre in northwest Calgary on the morning of January 10, 2016:

"Where's my hair?"

"Why are there fluorescent lights?"

"I'm on morphine?"

I managed to croak out a scratchy "Nurse?" that equally strained my voice and my ability to communicate at all. Instantly, a woman appeared at the door.

"Good. You're awake "

"Where's my hair?" I responded.

"Let me get the doctor," she replied as she vanished from my maladjusted sight back into the medical white light of the hallway.

A slender, dark-haired man in a white coat, tan slacks, and loafers strolled through the door. A considerate and subtle smile belied the seriousness of his tone and overall demeanour as he introduced himself. He explained that I had undergone emergency brain surgery.

The previous night I had been dropped off at the Sheldon M. Chumir Health Centre in non-responsive distress after an assault that resulted in a right epidermal haematoma, revealed by a CT scan preformed post haste on site. Following the scan, I was rushed to Foothills for an urgent craniotomy for evacuation of the haematoma, where I awoke with a fresh scar and shaved head.

The information given was able to answer the questions of where I was and why I was there. It also shed a thin beam of dim light onto the events of the night before, though they were yet to be fully illuminated. It would be much later before light would be shed by third-person accounts. There, however, remained two questions that needed answers.

"Where's my hair?"

"We had to shave your head to operate." Then the doctor added, "It was swept up and discarded," as though he thought I wanted to keep it or hoped for it to be reattached somehow.

"Where's my phone?"

The second question was in part concern for the status and whereabouts of my personal property as I had no recollections of what had exactly occurred that led to these drugged, shaven, and fluorescent moments of bewildered awakening. It was also a knee-jerk reaction to the implications of the situation and how it would undoubtedly negatively affect the likelihood of starting my new job at ten o'clock the next morning.

I had been hired to be a member of the opening brigade of an izakaya in the Mission area of Calgary. Leading up to this rare and interesting opportunity, I had spent hours online, researching history, menus, and methods. I had watched hours of videos on butchery and yakitori techniques. I wanted a base-level understanding before stepping out of the familiar comfort of Euro-centric cuisine into the unknown realm of a Japanese izakaya.

It was with this in mind, after having had the location of my clothes and phone revealed, that I made my first phone call from that recovery bed in Foothills. I called the chef of what would become a top-fifty restaurant in Canada to explain why I would not be able to be there for opening day. After expressing his shock and concern for my predicament, he explained that he understood and asked that I keep him informed, adding that if there was anything he could do to let him know. Then he asked if I had called my family. I hadn't. I had called him first. He let out a half a chuckle before ending the conversation with "Thanks for thinking of me. Now call your family."

Prior to writing the following I had had to text my father. I needed to confirm that after I called him, he arrived the next day. I was wrong. Obviously, he would not have arrived that day, as there was simply no time to make it to Halifax or Moncton to catch an improbably convenient direct flight to Calgary whilst reliving the frightful panic of hearing that your youngest son had suffered the malevolence of severe head trauma.

Notwithstanding is the irrefutable, undeniable fact that I didn't call him. My dear cousin did. I called her and don't remember. In fact, my memory of those hours is spotty. Was I there for hours? Was I there for days? What was my nurse's name again and why exactly did I have a nurse, anyway?

"Where's my hair?"

Oh, yeah. Now I remember.

It was only the immediate that mattered then. In a way, it is all that matters still. I remember one day my cousin and dad helped me out of the hospital bed, away from the institutionally lit recovery room and into the elevator. I'd like to think we walked unscathed through the myriad questions and concerns as the hum of fluorescent lights turned into the rays of the sun, beaming onto my surgically shaven head. The cool breeze caused my fresh new scar to pull tight, nerve cells cringing in relapsing fetal instinct, as the sound of sliding doors closed behind me. We crossed the threshold from the hospital to the parking lot, winter whispering a chill into the comforting kiss of the sun.

I still cannot recall when or how I arrived at my apartment, let alone the details of how I left.

"Why does it matter where my hair is?"

7
Events Come to Light

Saturday, January 9, 2016, was a momentous day.

Drug lord Joaquín El Chapo Guzmán had been recaptured earlier that day in Los Mochis. A presidential hopeful named Donald Trump held a rally in South Carolina, much to the chagrin of the rationally minded. And I? I got my ass kicked outside Vern's, a favoured watering hole in downtown Calgary.

I was in attendance to support friends who were playing a gig. Vern's low-lit basement feel sets a fantastic tone for the myriad punk and metal shows that occur on a small stage before a wall of cracked and chipped cymbals. The latter genre was what had brought me there that night. I was to treat my ears to the jarring brutality of death grind as delivered by Morley's own Dethgod. I had known the guys in the band for years at this point and seldom missed a show. I was also there to support other local bands, Ye Goat Herd Gods being one.

My support of local musicians often manifests itself through my buying of merch—patches, T-shirts, and the like. In fact, the last thing I remember of that night was buying a Ye Goat Herd Gods patch for my battle jacket. It was still in my pocket when I awoke in the hospital the next day.

The night was to be my last free Saturday of the foreseeable future as I was to start a new job the next Tuesday and my weekends would be lost to the restaurant industry once more. This meant that I should probably make it a good one. My new vaporizer packed with weed and a cash-thick wallet stuffed into my back pocket, I walked down the stairs into Vern's, where I proceeded to shoot Jack Daniels and swill down pints. I would step out the backdoor with this friend or that for a cigarette, a hoot, or both. Needless to say, as the night went on, I got considerably more twisted. This was not uncommon in the least and no one thought anything of it. A lot of metal shows at various venues in Calgary are blurry memories and a new black T-shirt in the morning. I have about sixty band shirts—but I digress.

The visiting band was a two-piece from Edmonton, a drummer and a tech-savvy guitarist with a black metal sound that resonated disharmonic loops through a processor. Three guys had followed them down from Edmonton, presumably for support, though they didn't seem the type to enjoy such intense musical expression as would be found there that night. Something about them must have rubbed me the wrong way as I recall making snide and dismissive remarks to them, which wasn't characteristic of me, even when intoxicated. It turned out I was not alone in my instinctive distaste for these three strangers, as they were bounced by the owner after a series of rude and disrespectful actions. They trashed a merch booth and were belligerent to some of the young women in attendance, one of whom was the girlfriend of the vocalist of the fourth band on the bill that night.

For months that followed that night, when I was going to therapy daily to recuperate from another craniotomy, I would struggle fruitlessly to recall what exactly had happened. As my last recollection of dealings with those responsible for me having been hospitalized was that of being uncharacteristically assertive, I could only assume that I had instigated with a series of drunken insults and deprecating jokes. It wasn't entirely unheard of for me to become boisterous if the brown liquor took hold the wrong way, but I'm not prone to be degrading to others. That behaviour is uncharacteristic, particularly to strangers. Still, there was every reason to believe that I had gotten "tough-guy drunk" and had bitten off more than I could chew, which is surprisingly little, to be honest. I figured I likely got into someone's face, real close and personal, then began mouthing off at an obnoxious volume. Profanity and boozy breath bellowed forth from me to them until they simply could no longer tolerate it and escalated the situation, kicking my ass for being stupid enough to antagonize.

I was certain that I had gotten beat down on account of my big mouth and felt a degree of embarrassment for it.

I talked to my psychiatrist about it as well as my father. The overall response from anyone was not to worry about it. Whatever led to the assault was neither here nor there. All that mattered was that I was alive and improving. I accepted that I was likely at fault, and that it would have been entirely avoidable had I governed myself wisely instead of becoming a loud, drunken ass.

The months went by and the notion that I had brought this frivolously on myself tacitly lingered as I continued to attend my various therapeutic appointments and adjust to new challenges as they arose. I wasn't going out too much at this point, partially because I often had appointments in the early morning and partially out of a bit of fear that something might happen. After all, things can always get worse.

The idea that I had, for no justifiable reason, been the cause of all the trials and tribulations I was navigating wafted about, filling the air I breathed with toxic self-blame. So much of my devotion to therapy was secretly penance for the crime I had committed against myself, a devastating failure to use better sense. I had created a version of the story wherein I was the exact kind of drunken douche that I normally would avoid and detest from a distance of better company. I had said and done this and that, none of which I could remember, and had caused the situation to escalate to excess. Uncharacteristically, but not unheard of, I had been the fuse, the catalyst that had brought about my discomforts. It had been my fault. Worse still was the notion that the whole ordeal was unnecessary and entirely avoidable. I got my head kicked in for nothing. I was in daily therapy and reliving past trauma as a result of getting my ass kicked for nothing. I was just another statistical drunk who'd picked a fight for no goddamn reason outside a bar in whatever city for nothing—and lost. More than embarrassed, I was ashamed.

When people would ask what had happened, I would tell them the truth to the best of my knowledge. The only information that was at my disposal was from my medical file, which only detailed the results. There was no ready information as to what had exactly occurred beyond my getting in a fight and being hospitalized with an epidermal hematoma as a result of losing badly. There was no police report as charges were never laid, cops were never involved. I had no significant memory of the events that I could have related to the police anyway, so it would likely have been chalked up as just another bar fight on another Saturday night in downtown Calgary. Besides, I was too focused on healing, on getting back to where I was before that night. I wanted to forget about it and push forward, despite the anger I harboured toward those who were responsible, even though I had no idea who they were. I couldn't remember at all what had happened, including who had done it. It somehow didn't seem worth it to delve deeper into who and why; my cerebral focus was needed elsewhere. I needed to focus on therapy. The challenge of basic math, matching shapes, and recognizing patterns was taxing enough without added the hurdles of police reports, investigations, and possible court appearances. I was already overwhelmed as I again familiarized myself with the common and mundane tasks of everyday life.

So, for a while, I had little information to share beyond that which I was given by doctors and therapists, which only pertained to the extent of my injuries and recovery methods. Of the fight that night and its aftermath I only knew that two members of Dethgod had intervened, which saved my life. I also knew that a young blonde woman drove me to the hospital. I have only a vague recollection of her presence, the memory has no visual details.

It was decided that she, not my friends, should drive me to the hospital a few blocks away. If you are wondering why my friends didn't drive me, I will tell you this: They are from Morley and the idea of natives bringing an unconscious white guy recently beaten up would not be well received at a hospital in Calgary as graciously as a tiny blonde woman doing the same thing. It was a wise decision, as the guys would have been scrutinized by the police on duty at the hospital on that Saturday night. They would have just thought her my girlfriend and approached with less suspicion and more sympathy.

Eventually I would start stepping out at night, going again to bars and shows. The notion of going to Vern's again still made me apprehensive—not out of concern that anything would happen but that being there might trigger disquieting memories to surface from out of the darkness of brain trauma.

I had already gone to a major show at Mac Hall and survived. I had been to this bar and that without incident. My social life was coming back to life, and I was a little flabbergasted by the support and respect I was receiving from so many in the metal scene. Friends would make inquiries and offer well-wishes. I had people looking out from me whenever I went out, my best interest sincerely in mind. I thought it was just the usual kindness and support that you could expect from friends and acquaintances after surgery and rehabilitation. It was that, but also something more, as I would find out soon after walking into the Lord Nelson bar for a Mystifier show. I was standing in front of the stage for under a minute before I realized who I was standing beside. I turned quickly to my left and, with unabashed enthusiasm, said, "You drove me to the hospital! Thank you!"

I immediately expressed my gratitude for what she had done for me, explaining that she had helped save my life. I told her that for the rest of her life I would be in her debt. Then she thanked me. I paused and looked at her puzzled, not sure what she could possibly have to thank me for. I was just a drunken ass that had gotten beaten into the intensive care unit and likely a source of much stress and inconvenience that night. Not to mention a plausible bloody mess in her car. My confusion evident, she asked me if I remembered what happened that night. I admitted that I had essentially no memory of the night and asked her to tell me what she could.

That which she had to tell me would fill in a significant span of missing time, information of the events that led up to my suffering the head trauma. I still to this day, five years later, have no personal recollection of the events. To be honest, even what she told me about that night is not as clear a memory as I would like. The years that have passed have taken some of the details with them, but to the best of my knowledge, the events unfolded as follows.

Shortly after the three unwanted guests were ousted from Vern's for their various misdeeds and transgressions, she went up the stairs to have a cigarette on the sidewalk out front. I would not be long behind her, also wanting a cigarette. When I got outside, I was greeted with a disturbing scene. Those three guys had not left the area and had her surrounded as she stood against the wall. They were assailing her with insults and profanity, threateningly looming over her five-foot-two frame. I interjected. Apparently, I was calm and collected when I approached. She told me I was "chill" as I strolled toward them, politely asking them to calm down as their aggression toward a ninety-pound woman was excessive and unnecessary. Seeing as I had already been rude and antagonistic, I soon found the aggression of one of these cowardly bastards directed at me. No

Skull Fragments

longer looming over a lone woman barraging her with threats and insults, he stood toe-to-toe with me, cursing menacingly. He clearly had no intention of leaving with his friends without further incident, so I made a snap decision in response to his threats. That decision wasn't to throw the first punch. It wasn't to walk away—how could I in those circumstances/ I opted instead to pluck his ball cap off his head, fling it nonchalantly into the street, and suggest that he "Fuck off, find his hat, and get hit by a cab."

It is at this point that he punched me in the face.

She told me I "came back swinging," but how she said it gave me the impression it was an ineffective and unskilled counter. The other two had stepped away from her by then and one of them stuck me hard from behind. I stumbled over a cement parking brick, the kind that prevents a car from getting too close to the sidewalk. I hit the ground with force, my head crashing against the asphalt of Stephen Avenue. I was instantly unconscious.

They then started to put the boots to me.

They likely would have continued had my friends not come out just in time to intervene. Two of them got beaten to a pulp as the third took off down the street. I was lying on the asphalt, eyes rolled to white and body twitching as tremours of trauma and pain ricocheted through my brain.

By the end of our conversation at the Lord Nelson we both had tears in our eyes. She thanked me again, for coming to her rescue. Had I not come out when I did, she was not sure what may have happened. They may have physically attacked her as all evidence would indicate that as the next step in such a volatile situation. Her boyfriend also thanked me. He was beyond impressed that I had stood up for her when she was in danger, a sentiment echoed by his bandmates and others. All the respect and support I had been receiving made sense after that. People, mere acquaintances, coming up to me at shows or bars and expressing their concern for what had happened finally added up. I was, to an extent, a hero of sorts.

I had come to the aid of a woman in distress. I had put myself very much in harm's way for a reason that one could say was very much justifiable, if not even noble.

The knowledge that I was mistaken as to what had actually occurred that night, that I had suffered all that I had for no reason beyond being a drunken idiot that couldn't keep his mouth shut, was a shot in the arm. The shame and embarrassment dissipated—regarding the circumstances, at least. Thereafter, whenever I felt discouraged and disinterested in progressing, I had another new source of motivation. My actions had potentially saved someone from a similar if not more devastating outcome. As rough a road as I may have been on as a result of that night, I took great comfort in knowing that she was unscathed. It empowered me to know that I had acted with a bravery of sorts; that my actions may have prevented a greater tragedy. That she was fine, and I was on the mend made it worth it in a way.

It gave me confidence.

8
Don't Let Them Win

Don't let them win. Throughout my therapy I would repeat this in my head. Don't let them win.

Don't let them win, as I learned to recognize patterns and shapes, as I reignited the synaptic candle of basic math. When I would awaken in the morning and my first taste of conscious life would bedazzle my palate with confusion and disbelief, lingering tannins of melancholy that whispered fragility. While filling in a calendar with the dates and times of unabated trips to Sheldon Chumir for more therapy. Every fucking time I wanted to give up: stop trying, stop fighting, stop this incalculable world from spinning about.

Don't let them win. Those fucking cowardly drunkards that put me in the hospital may have never given the night a passing thought beyond the point of healing from their wounds. They probably headed back to Edmonton and shrugged off the night as another toss-up shit show as black eyes faded, and busted ribs mended from my friends effective retaliation. No hospital necessary. Life unchanged, they got to walk away not unscathed, just uninhibited.

This idea upsets me. This idea I used to fuel me daily as I would walk down 4th Street from 15th Avenue upwards of three times daily for therapy, whether it was psychological in the morning or occupational in the late afternoon, I would repeat to myself before a mirror, transfixed by the jagged, arching scar on my head, "Don't let them win." Then I would head out to conquer. Being a mere survivor wasn't good enough. They would not win. I couldn't allow it.

I still chant that to myself at times, this empowering mantra that is words and a vision. Every time my limbic system glitches, misfires, and I respond irrationally I find myself repeating, "Don't let them win." Still to this day, over four and a half years later, "Don't let them win" reverberates when all I want is for everything to fuckin' stop.

I am beginning to realize that I've never stopped telling myself that. The words ricochet in infinite tangents in all I do. Sometimes I'm listening and sometimes I'm not, but in the end, I've always heard and will always hear those words breaking the silence, drowning out the cacophony.

Don't let them win.

9

REHABILITATING MISE EN PLACE

Months of therapy and rehabilitation had run their course. A panel review of my file, my test scores, and overall progress was conducted at Sheldon Chumir. All my therapists and doctors were in attendance to primarily discuss the results of four and a half hours of neuropsychological testing I had completed at Foothills.

This was part of a "back-to-work" plan with which the CAR (Community Accessible Rehabilitation) team had been expertly helping me. A video conference with the neurologist who oversaw my care at the Foothills Brain Injury Clinic primarily focused on my scores on all the tests I had taken. The results of the sixteen tests of various cognitive domains were examined, accompanied with input and consultation. I had scored in the average-to-high-average scale, even topping out in the superior level on a couple of tests.

One that I did struggle with was mentioned and some discussion was had. It was a test of executive function to assess the flexibility of my thoughts when it came to problem-solving. I scored a low average on the Wisconsin Card Sorting Test on account of a weak start; I was uncertain how to perform the task, how to preserve appropriate responses to challenges. The young woman who had tested me made note that once I figured it out, I excelled beyond average, though it took me a hot minute to get there. My psychiatrist, always encouraging, said that if I took the test again, she believed I would have no issues. The panel agreed.

In particular, they referenced my score on the executive function test for word fluency. The D-KEFS (Delis-Kaplan Executive Function System) for word fluency would be my highest score: very superior phonemic fluency. I was informed in that meeting that I had scored within the top three percentile. Everyone was very impressed and proud, but I was humble when I explained it was luck. After all, the test had me saying as many words as possible that fit a certain criteria in a given time frame.

The criteria I was assigned was to cite as many fruits and vegetables as I could. After nearly two decades in professional kitchens, it wasn't a challenge. I explained that all I had to do was think of a produce order sheet as I listed off examples in alphabetical order. Had the topic been different, I would not have scored as high, but that was inconsequential. It had been decided that I should return to work part time.

Obviously, I would opt to re-enter the kitchen, though at a less demanding capacity. My neuropsychological assessments had given positive results in various domains of executive function, and visuospatial and fine motor skills. I felt fairly confident that I was again ready to don a white coat and commit to cuisine. I was admittedly keenly aware that there would be challenges. Even my assessment from Foothills stipulated that I could possibly "experience difficulties in more complex real-world environments that are more stimulating." Multitasking skills, in particular, were mentioned. The report then cited a "noisy kitchen" as such an environment. Undeterred, I sought employment part time in a reputable restaurant. It was all I knew and far less daunting than exploring a new career path.

The job at the izakaya I was to begin before I found myself in the hospital after an emergency craniotomy was no longer available. It had been months and, to his credit, the chef had held a place for me as long as he could. I would later find out that it was likely for the best as the job would have been a rough gig, to put it nicely.

The job I had left just prior to the assault that hospitalized me had been supportive of me during my recuperation and would continue to be so. My former chef, and friend, was able to set me up with a part-time gig at a small French bistro a mere block from home. An award-winning and established restaurant in the Beltline district of Calgary, it provided me with exactly what I needed to get back into the swing of things. The hours were enough to cover my expenses without over burdening me during that early phase of my recovery. Though a handful of my friends and family thought I would start smaller, like a dishwasher in a pub, I jumped back in at a more demanding depth. Even the *garde manger* position in a fine dining setting would be enough of a challenge to push me to the uttermost limit of my cognitive acuity, often beyond.

I still recall hearing the chef yelling my name in the middle of service on a busy night, when my brain would short-circuit and shut down. My catatonic stupor disrupted by the shouts, I would come back into the moment perplexed and disassociated, not entirely sure what I was to be doing or even where exactly I was. I would struggle to remember what ingredients were needed to create a beef tartar. I would forget a dessert on a bill or lose track of the timing on entrées. This didn't happen constantly, but enough to cause me frustration and some degree of embarrassment. I had been hyped up a bit to the chef. My friend had spoken so highly of me that there had been no need for an interview. I was embarrassed when I fell behind or made a mistake, more so when I would completely shut down. I was not accustomed to having a busy kitchen so overwhelm me and found it discouraging.

It wasn't how I remembered it, not at all.

I remembered being efficient and focused, nearly beyond reproach. I was better than this stumbling, distracted, and forgetful mess I had become. I was better, once upon a time. I had to improve. I had to work harder. I had to attain at least a semblance of the skill and ability I once possessed. The brain injury I suffered wouldn't rob me of all I had worked and sacrificed to achieve. Those who attacked me would not take cuisine from me. I needed to succeed again, even if it meant starting from nearly scratch.

There is no denying that a degree of patience and understanding was involved on the parts of the chef, sous chef, and owners of the bistro. I had made my situation very clear before I started there. The chef that had arranged the job for me had also referred to my injury previously but left the particulars for me to explain. There were times that I had to be reminded of this or that, times I needed to be pushed more assertively and times when my actions caused noticeable frustration within management, but I was never let go. In fact, as the business began to get busier, my hours increased. With more business comes more prep, so my responsibilities also increased. This all fortunately occurred incrementally, at a rate I was able to manage. Multi-tasking and time management began to improve, as did my focus and confidence. I was able to again memorize recipes and properly anticipate the required *mise en place*. I appreciated the patience shown me during my recuperation to this point and I let them know as much. I was beginning to feel like I was on the right track and building solid momentum toward my goal of reaching the same level of culinary skill and experience I had known before. Content and motivated, I was confident that the bistro gig, with its classic French menu and small, devoted staff, would continue to be a spring of opportunity for me to re-establish my skills, re-install my abilities, and remember the knowledge I garnered over years.

Unfortunately, my hours would be cut for a variety reasons, none of which were a reflection on my performance. This made it fiscally unreasonable for me to stay on board. I was again on the job hunt. The various neuroplasticity exercises that exist within professional kitchen work had been of great help. Processes involving repetitive tasks, multi-tasking, and time-management skills were all fired up in a synaptic light show of executive function. My efficiency in matters à la carte had returned to a greater degree and I was feeling confident, strong in my conviction that I could again run the line and manage staff. I would apply primarily to sous chef positions as a means not to re-establish my career but to further my progressive cerebral coherence. I needed the extra responsibility and pressure if I was to continue to push through the mire of my brain trauma and return to the life I had known.

The added challenges that came with a sous chef gig would easily provide just enough to keep me developing all that I had temporarily lost, the momentum needed to not just continue but accelerate. My brain was to be engorged with the neurological stimuli mandated to rewire previous connections. The framework was there, just damaged and dysfunctional. The time at the bistro did a lot of the early heavy lifting in regard to recuperating my acuity, but the time had come for more detailed and demanding work to begin.

I got my opportunity for it at an upscale burger joint in Bridgeland. It was not open yet, so I was able to get in from the very outset and put my problem-solving and multitasking skills to the test almost immediately.

Only a few weeks into being open the kitchen was being bombarded with chits and was clamouring to maintain a near clockwork precision under my command. While orchestrating the flow of the kitchen, governing the timing, and dictating the execution of duties of the entire kitchen, I began to feel like my old self again. It was invigorating. It was reassuring.

Further reassurance came from the chef. He told me he was impressed with how well I oversaw the rush of guests that had arrived from downtown offices at the end of the business day. He said I could clearly run a kitchen and asked if there was anything he could teach me. I explained that my administrative skills were lacking. My math skills had been hampered by what had happened to the extent that I had had to learn relatively basic math again under the supervision of the CAR team. He assured me that he would show me the ins and outs. He also expressed his contentment in knowing that I was able to oversee, to his specifications, the operations of his brigade in his absence. Then he left for the day, leaving me at the helm—a confidence boost that was as appreciated as it was needed.

Another dose of reassurance came at the end of the rush when the owner informed me that one of the guests wanted to talk with me if I was available. I was and it very much fell within the scope of my titular responsibilities to converse with guests from time to time. I consented to have the guests come up to the kitchen doorway to speak with me about whatsoever they wished. I was expecting either accolades or complaints, as they were the usual motives for a guest to wish to speak to the chef. I reckoned this would be a test of my humility or patience respectively. My demeanour would need to remain professional and courteous if I was to interact with the person, whether the theme of the conversation was positive or negative—a challenge to my tired and distracted brain, though not a terribly daunting one, all things considered.

As the guest approached, I quickly realized that the nature of their desire to speak with me was not about the dining experience they had had. The guest was my former occupational therapist. A charming, intelligent, and attractive blonde woman was suddenly standing in front of me with a smile on her face, jovial eyes dancing behind her glasses. She stood nearly toe to toe with me as her hand touched my arm, lingering there a moment in a gentle display of empathy. Perhaps her hand also lingered for a little extra stability, as she was just on the friendly side of tipsy. She was enthusiastic about seeing me. Her smile beaming, her eyes dancing, she told me how thrilled she was to see me calling the line, running the kitchen.

When I had been under her care at Sheldon Chumir, she had devised an exercise to evaluate my ability to focus and multitask. She had researched how calling a line works, how a kitchen runs. It was necessary to research as she had no familiarity with work in a restaurant. The exercise she staged was for me to respond to "orders" as she called them out, including pickups and modification. This was done not in the clinic on the fifth floor but in the coffee shop on the ground floor of the hospital. She knew very well that I would have marginal issues with such an exercise in the pristine and calm hospital examination room, so the test was conducted amidst the hustle and clamour of the coffee shop. The concern regarding potential "difficulties in more complex real-world environments" needed to be explored to some degree if she were to accurately assess my condition and rate of rehabilitation.

She reminded me with glee and genuine pride of that exercise she had put such effort into arranging. To witness me doing practically the exact exercise in my post-therapeutic life, only far more complex, in the restaurant that occupied the ground floor of her building, was an unexpected and pleasant surprise. Before returning to her table and who I assumed was her date, I listened intently as she expressed her admiration for how devoted I was to my therapy and her pride in how far I had come in such a short time. She specialized in individuals with multiple brain injuries and had months prior told me how exceptional I was to be able to apply myself as I do. It had impressed her at the time.

Once again impressed by my tenacity, she imparted words of encouragement and well-wishing before a brief embrace and departure. I was left feeling accomplished and confident that things would steadily improve for me in accordance with the work I put in. With a faint feeling of triumphant achievement, I returned to work.

My time at the burger joint would come to a halt upon my dismissal. The emotional turbulence by which I was beleaguered after significant damage to my frontal lobe had begun increasingly to create problems until one day my temper flared and I behaved tyrannically and without censor.

The following day I was let go. My presence had become a source of discomfort for the front-of-house staff and the servers had strong reservations about working with me lest my temper and aggression become directed at them. As much as the technical and managerial aspects of my job were relatively on point, my emotional fluctuations were still too problematic for me to handle the full spectrum of responsibilities required of me.

After I was let go, most of the kitchen quit. They supported and respected me more than the chef, whom they held partially accountable for my dismissal as I was overworked and often picking up his slack.

In the end I found comfort in the discovery of a degree of limitation. I knew where the wall was, the boundary hindering my progression. I also knew what I was capable of if I put in the work necessary and would commence doing so forthwith. I was no longer in a place in life where I could allot time and energy to the vacuous nature of defeat. It was time for a new mandate. I would not lose. I would win or I would learn. I would gather the positive experiences and lessons from my time at that burger joint in Bridgeland and incorporate them into my outlook, my modus operandi.

10
BAD BRAIN DAYS

A "bad brain day" is a generalized term I use when my cerebral cortex seems to be exceedingly out of sorts. I apply it to occasions of psychological, emotional, or cognitive distress that impede my daily life.

Though rare, these extreme synaptic malfunctions are exhausting and drain me of vitality. Those three aspects of my psyche are usually affected simultaneously, though they vary by degrees each time. Confused by warrantless anger, I become depressed and ashamed, for example. Furthermore, each area of affect has what would basically constitute sub-regions of affect. Forthwith I will delve into this anomaly that assails me at most unexpected times.

The aforementioned affliction isn't new, in the relative since. I didn't acquire this instability as a result of my most recent brain injury over five years ago. At least I don't believe I did. The mood swings and instability of my early teenage years seem to have the same flavour. There is also the steady line of consecutive girlfriends that expressed, though in drastically different tones, concern or frustration about my mood, outlook, or general demeanour on any given day insofar as it was unpredictable. "I never know each morning which Len I'm going to get," one had put it. This leads me to believe that I have always suffered these paradoxical shifts, at least since the time of my first encephalic trauma. The second brain injury only exasperated the matter, grey and white inclusive.

Terrible plays on words aside, we are all subject to bad days from time to time. Those wrong-side-of-the bed awakenings into a realm of familiarity blown askew by winds of mishap and misfortune wherein setbacks seem to accumulate ad nauseam, the echoing consequences of one mild calamity ebbing into the next in succession and leaving dwindling hope of stabilization in its wake. A moment's reprieve is often all that is needed to regain control of the day's events. A breath of fresh air or a step back from the maelstrom of reactionary thought can usher forth a balancing of the scales and allow the mind to again perceive and progress with clarity. However, if the brain is the source of the calamity, then the hope of such a reprieve is nullified to a great extent. Bad luck and poor planning don't figure into it. They also can neither account for nor be circumvented to adjust to the apparent reality. When the very tool you need to repair, improve, or remedy a situation is faulty and failing, it feels as though you are cut adrift in the overwhelming mire and turbulence of a chaotic procession. The inner monologue becomes an incessant diatribe drowning out self-assurance's soothing whispers. Trapped inside one's own head, enveloped in pandemonium of thought, the physical self and world at large take on a more challenging tone. Everything becomes more difficult. Manoeuvring through obstacles that were once familiar and of no consequence one's goals are based on temporal proximity, having traded the future for the instantaneous through bare necessity.

Weeks have elapsed since I first began exploring this subject. In the interim there were days clearly infected and affected by the phenomenon, which had manifested in one way or another. The three-day stint of inexplicable predisposed anger stands out. It was as though a predatory inclination toward rageful responses was being propagated from within, encouraged and spurred by an unreasonable and unreasoning voice wafting up from the darker recesses of my mind. The nearly ceaseless yattering of hasty presumptions and ill-gotten conclusions had me continuously on edge. I was aware enough only to be able to rein in my misguided and delusional outrage lest I erupt inappropriately, yet I could not fully squelch the fire and fury that rumbled beneath the surface. I would endure, but not without making a spectacle of myself one night after regretfully imbibing in excess, ignoring better judgement. Anger and frustration on gales of cheap vodka and economy beer lashed about my living room late one night. My roommate, whom I had awoken with my outburst, gave me a wide berth the following morning as I cleaned the incidental wreckage of my baseless fury. I felt shame. It was flavoured with the disappointment of my actions and the confusion of their inexplicable nature.

The effects of preventing myself from flying off the handle at each and every irritation may have exacerbated the mental exhaustion I felt. That fatigue of the mind is not unheard of as it is, so perhaps the two are unrelated. I sometimes suffer from extended periods of impeded cognizance for hours on end. Conversely, this can lead to frustration. Occasionally it's a cycle, one neurological dysfunction feeding into the other in a closed-circuit disharmony over which I often feel nearly powerless. Draining and depressing, I am rendered in shades duller and more faded.

When the cognizance and cerebral capabilities are at low swing, at their worst, it is a somnambulist's nightmare. Immediate surroundings and situations, though clear, convey their meaning with notable less assurance, less insistence. My senses decipher through a decelerating haze. Even the familiar and common become shackled and stifled by an inhibited cortical registration and response. Slower to recognize, register, and respond, I watch from within as routine tasks are temporarily more demanding of concentration than the previous day.

My brain, already hampered and retrograding, can perceive these inhibited interactions with my environment but do nothing about them. The irony of the situation isn't lost, but it garners no

Len Roach

mirth or humour of any kind as I struggle through broken lenses to better discern fine details blurred and out of focus. Possessing the awareness of what is happening, though appreciated, adds a facet of duality to my mere existence. Although my acuity for the immediate is faltering at these times I am able to witness it as if a spectator. My mind's eye taken notice of every moment of slowed response and tentative choice like watching a child's first step or a fledgling leaving the nest on its maiden flight, necessity and hesitation fast in hand. Luckily, I have been blessed with the ability to retain enough self-awareness to address the issue or at least refer to it among friends and colleagues so as to provide a length of slack to counter the missteps and miscalculations that may arise. Mirthless and relatively detached I plod onward through the hours waiting for abatement, reprieve and the return of my full faculties. The knowledge and memory of my customary and preferred state of mind resonating through the whole ordeal, I am left feeling incomplete and lessened. Powerless to prevent the unheralded arrival of such periods of cerebral struggle I can only wade passively within those muddied waters for the languid storm to pass and cling with bittersweet nostalgia to recollections of a time before such occurrence would besiege me.

11
The Impending Plausible Retrograde

Just moments ago, I looked up chronic traumatic encephalopathy (CTE). Before today I didn't know what the name for the condition was, though I was certain it had one.

Over the last four years, since the second brain surgery, I have been introduced to several new terms. I would, at long last, find or be given names to the events, the conditions, and effects that have plagued me incessantly since my teen years. The addition of definitive terminology to better understand and explore the endless theatre of mystery that is my damaged and hindered brain was like an instruction manual in a language I would need to learn on the fly. Multi-syllable, Latin-centric medical jargon would register briefly before falling out of the reach of retention into the great dark expanse of things forgotten. What they defined I remember because I live it: limbic system, ABI/TBI, and paraxial epidermal hematoma, for example. Some things I have forgotten the name of or what they are in reference to and need to research again from time to time. Others I may have outright avoided, as I didn't want to think about them. I didn't want to name the devil that whispers such dreadful premonitions. I had my own internal Schrödinger's cat of existential crisis. With all the stress and struggle already permeating days on end, I couldn't allot that devil the dignity of acknowledgment.

Today, while choking back a dart and listening to opus 129 "Rage over a Lost Penny," I opened the box for a quick peek. Chronic traumatic encephalopathy is a neurodegenerative disease that causes severe and irreparable damage to the brain. It is a result of repeated head injuries. It can take years for the symptoms to manifest, and usually does. I fear it. The idea, the very fucking notion of it, fills me with dreadful thoughts. An anxious and apprehensive trepidation of a plausible future when the confusion and dysfunction will return like ruthless offspring of torments once thought conquered if not fully vanquished. I've been avoiding it. Like a child with comfort pulled tight over his head, eyes shut and muttering mantras of disbelief about the presumed monster under the bed. I couldn't muster the courage to look into what lead to the death of Derek Boogaard of Saskatoon, a twenty-eight-year-old NHL player whose accidental overdose led to the discovery of CTE. I have heard of other cases of athletes in physical sports suffering from long-term effects of ABI/TBI. I was unable to watch *Concussion* (2015, Columbia Pictures), starring Will Smith as Dr. Bennet Omalu for the same reason I couldn't previously explore the subject. I wasn't willing to add to the struggle by worrying about a possible future negative event, so I buried my head in the sand. I tried not to think about it, pushing the thought away as best I could. The idea is still so intensely disheartening that it takes the air out of the room, the warmth within gets colder and I begin to wane. I felt it necessary to stay just out of arm's reach of the beast, to keep my mind focused as I sprang from thought to thought away from the fear that, in my periphery, stalks and conspires. The more immediate troubles were in much need of tending so the frightful prospect of CTE had to wait to be named, to be acknowledged, to have its day in the spotlight. Thus, it is with reluctance and hesitation that I am writing this. Having been actively avoiding the topic all these years, I have programmed my brain with Pavlovian intent to derail such trains of thought. Like a dog at the table begging for scraps, it whines, hoping for a bit of reassurance or a jovial recollection. I must ignore the distractions flung out of the darkness in the back of my mind and acquiesce to the need to face that fear I have just today discovered indeed has a name.

Chronic traumatic encephalopathy is a four-tiered disease that progresses menacingly over the years. Memory loss, explosivity, and spatial dysfunction are symptoms. All who suffer have had suicidal moments. Depression, aggression, and variant mood swings. Executive dysfunctions disinhibit. How bleak and futile does the world become as dementia consumes your final days.

Becoming again forgetful, moody, depressed, and angry is a concept that paralyzes me for an instant of nauseating panic. The statistical evidence of self-harm and suicide associated with the disease alone is a Houdini punch to the heart. I fear a future that could be waiting. I imagine myself again as I was just after the accident or just after having my head kicked in. I imagine a return to that disorientation while in familiar settings, a return of the overwhelming chimes and trumpets of emotional delusion and strife. I imagine a regression back into the bleak hours of self-hating solitude and disdain for a life fraying at the edges. The notion that all the work I have done to repair and redeem my tattered mind could be undone in time is not only frightening but indeed heartbreaking. In that moment of nauseating panic, I find motivation and optimism absent, blotted out like a dark cloud passing before a waxing moon. Sometimes it lasts a few minutes; it is rarely an hour before I can divert my thoughts to something constructive or at least reassuring. I remind myself that all is well, in a relative sense. The cloud passes eventually, and the light shines again, just slightly brighter than before perhaps, though the shadows remain.

Always whispering in my ear is the same fear, that someday there would begin a regression of faculties, a retrograde through traumatic events of synaptic misfires. The self I had begun to accept and nurture morphing into the one I sought to leave behind. Haunted by the thought of persona and perspective relapsing into an epoch of my life in which perseverance was a miraculous feat. Taxing enough to recall, unfathomable to relive such days, the idea also motivates me. Like Charlie in *Flowers for Algernon* (Daniel Keyes. 1968 Bantam), when he realizes he faces the same fate as the lab mouse if he doesn't use all at his disposal to find an answer. I too must write these words and explore these fears because I can. Chronic traumatic encephalopathy is nothing more than a fear of a possible future, one of infinite possibilities. Today I can still write, work, and tend to my wants and needs with a clarity many in my situation have lost. Being cognizant and diligent is better than ignorant and fearful anyway. I should very well advise myself to delve deeper into the matter. Educate myself not just into readiness but empowerment, should the worst case come to be, and the clouds linger ever longer in days to come.

UPDATE: Two weeks after I wrote this I watched *Concussion*. I wept.

12
Factory Reset

Often, I become overwhelmed, the surging stimuli and the instantaneous responses colliding in a tidal bore of confusion. Ideas and experiences churn and froth behind my definitively expressive eyes. Grasping at anything to hold onto, I often become fixated on one notion or another, convincing myself of its validity. The event that made me angry, offended, upset, or whatnot is quickly and often mistakenly accepted as an absolute. Likewise, occurrences that bring me pleasure or delight become focal points of my attention in a singular fashion as I tend to omit any adjacent negativity. Whether positive or negative, my mood is set. My demeanour follows suit. I can remain disproportionately reactive for extended periods of time, often hours. Right or wrong, this rigid uncompromising stance is preferred over the swirling uncertainty of being overwhelmed.

Why shouldn't it be? After all, the following day I will awaken from a night's slumber without more than an inkling of the sentiment that had me so fired up. Through the night it is as though the very thing that had led to extremity of behaviour and perception hadn't happened in effective reality. The memory may remain in an abstract sense. I may recall vaguely what mechanisms were at work that caused me to have a reaction this way or that, but no recollection of why my reaction was so intense, so enveloping. Effectively the negativity that only a day prior had me incised or distraught would have been dispelled through the night. I am left feeling calm and refreshed, primarily regarding a particular source event or issue.

When I tell friends of this nightly "factory reset," they respond with envy. It must be nice not to carry your anger, your disappointment from one day into the next, to be free of that weighted burden and able to embrace anew the day ahead. It doesn't always happen, of course, just usually. When it does happen, it is nice. To have my frustrations, sorrows, disgust, and pain no longer shrouding my every thought is obviously preferred. However, for the ointment there is a fly, the thorn of the rose. It's not just the dark and negative emotions, thoughts, and actions that are scrubbed clean through the night. The joy and delight of yesterday's pleasantries are equally prone to redaction. It can be disheartening when the feelings and thoughts that bore forth optimism are absent from memory. Seemingly lost forever, those positive moments need to be replaced daily. Delicate orchids of the mind that could not withstand the night's subconscious upheavals. Every morning is greeted with so nearly a perfect balance of relief and regret for the absence of yesterday's anger and joy respectively that I might just as well have fallen fresh into my life and my predicament.

Of the more dire implications there is one that stands out. Risk assessment is hampered. The negativity that came from a particular situation or choice is needed to make the simple judgements to avoid repetitive mistakes. The more complete and comprehensive the understanding of what emotional reaction I had to an event, the better if I'm to avoid the same consequences. When the recollection is obscured so to is the lesson. The result is a series of faulty choices that could be more prudently contended with pre-emptively. Individuals and situations that justly caused alarm bells to ring clearly in my mind are too often pardoned with those that were legitimately blameless. I don't trust whether I was at fault or not for lack of cognizant recollection of how I was affected. Perhaps I was the problem, the catalyst. This can lead to me being manipulated. I can easily be gas-lit. That knowledge has left me to seek refuge in isolation. My pride doesn't want to lend time and opportunity to the possibility of being made a fool due to defaults in memory.

So nearly every day I awake to discover myself operating from a preset, core memory and my functions intact, for the most part. I find, willingly or not, new joys and frustrations to replace those that mysteriously vanished into the ether of dreams and nightmares.

13

Playing with a Full Deck

Over the years since that violent tussle outside a bar on 8th Avenue after a metal show, I have been living with the effects of severe cerebral trauma. There is not an easily perceived superficial or objectively obvious physical indication of the incident.

The surgery scars are behind my hairline and, thus, normally obscured. Even when my head is shaved into a mohawk, a hat is usually covering the scars. I often (perhaps too often) feel compelled to relate the nature of my unique situation to those I have just met, particularly if I have been drinking. Alcohol can have a sudden, divergent effect on me. I swerve from mere timid congeniality into realms that are melancholy or agitated, despondent or confused.

This propensity for the temperamental has left me saddled with a self-prescribing obligation to inform others of the deeper source of such potential shifts in demeanour—a well-practised and candid preamble, a disclaimer, if you would. Though I can quickly and with ease cite the basic gist of my predicament at the drop of a hat (yes, that was a callback), I have long considered an alternative that would perhaps save me and whoever I am in conversation with time.

My idea is simply to get business cards printed. I would always keep about a dozen cards on hand, particularly if I was planning on being in a crowded space and imbibing a few drinks. If on occasion I began to catch the notion that a shift of mood was coming about I could simply hand the card to whoever was in the area of affect and allow them to draw their own conclusions. An email would be printed on the back if they wished to contact me with any followup questions. The main body of the text would simply read something to the extent of:

> **Please Forgive**
> **Anything This Man**
> **Says or Does**
> He Has Two Brain Injuries

The problem with this plan is the slim chance I ever have a girlfriend again. That beautiful angel would receive like thirty a week.

14
HEAD SCARS AND HAIRCUTS

Prior to the events of September 9, 1991, I was well on my way to representing my affinity to metal music. I sported one from a small collection of T-shirts depicting the logos and album covers of Metallica, Iron Maiden, Metal Church, and others daily. And my hair was reaching shoulder length, though I was not fastidious in its upkeep.

Torn jeans and black T-shirts, long dark hair, and a Walkman bombarding my ears with thrash. I was a young metal head in junior high striving to be as cool as the older guys with their leather jackets and patch-covered denim vests, the cornerstone of the image being the long hair of musicians and fans alike. I refused to get mine cut and let it grow unabated.

When I was in the hospital in Moncton awaiting surgery to repair the fractured skull, I received from a thirteen-foot fall off that same high school I was attending in my metal shirts and torn jeans, my hair was progressively sprouting from my head. For months after I kept the blood-stained Ozzy "Bark at the Moon" baseball T that I wore the night of the fall before giving in to my mother for disposal in exchange for a deadly black leather motorcycle jacket. A step closer to my image goals, but I digress.

While I was in the hospital one of the nurses would tease me, a good-natured ribbing about how my hair would spread out like tendrils across the pillow as I slept. "Like sleeping beauty," she would say mischievously, a playful and kind smirk adorning her face, her eyes twinkling slightly within the border of subtle crow's feet. She would be present when the matter of how much of my hair I would like to keep was broached. Surgery would require that my head, from apex forward, be shaved fully. No choice in the matter. It was a question whether I wished to keep the length in the back. I had no interest in having a mullet and thought it more prudent to lose it all. I would merely have to start the whole process of growing it out again. No big deal. After all, I was still metal as all-hell on the inside, right?

After surgery, it was clear the deed had been done. Months upon months of growth had been shaved down to the scalp and, in lieu of dark brown tresses of wavy hair, I was crowned with a precise and blatant scar from temple to temple. Fifty-two surgical steel staples strafed in linear symmetry across my head just behind the hairline. The fresh incision protruded a bas relief of flesh and dried blood, segmented by that succession of staples that ached and itched ever so slightly. The follicles of my shorn cranium too seemed to tingle and itch, having not been so extensively exposed previously. Medicated and half-awake, I would instinctively seek out my locks every morning to no avail. That briefest moment of confusion would spur me awake before settling into the reality that my head was shaved and a scar of some significance and potency did now exist. The scar, as I was told a few days after surgery, gave me an appearance reminiscent of a baseball. This prospect I found amusing at the time, likely on account of the various drugs imbuing my intravenous with pleasantry and pain relief.

The scar would draw attention. The school-sanctioned remedy was that I would be allowed to cover my head with a ball cap while at school so I wouldn't distract anyone and wouldn't feel insecure. I believe I opted for a Metallica "Kill 'Em All" trucker cap; the mesh of that style allowed air flow, which was soothing to the wound still on the mend. I was able to shroud my unsightly scar from the world as my hair slowly grew back. Over the course of the next few years, I had again achieved a lengthy mane indicative of heavy metal music. What is more, I was far more attentive to it. I conditioned and combed, I air-dried, and I trimmed dead and split ends as needed. At one point while high on pills, I shaved an undercut, revealing a glimpse of the scar beneath. For the most part I let my hair hang free flowing, having never forgotten the bizarre appearance of my fully bald head. Even the undercut would grow in eventually. I was told I had beautiful hair and was proud to show it off, if not a bit arrogant, truth be told. Then one day during a mushroom trip I thought it reasonable to lob off my ponytail with a kitchen knife. This would require the corrective skills of a barber to make me at least presentable. I would not attempt to grow my hair so long again for years. I would get it cut and styled as anyone else might at a barbershop or salon.

So it was that I would find myself periodical in a chair before a mirror, a smock draped over me and a barber or stylist asking me how I would like my haircut. Whether it was an eighty-dollar session replete with scalp massage on Davie Street or a ten-buck quick trim at barber school on Broadway, there would undoubtedly be an inquiry about the scar. I could be on Commercial Drive in Vancouver or Main Street in Amherst, Nova Scotia. It didn't matter. Whoever was welding the scissors and clippers would ask how it was I came to have such a pronounced scar. I would, for my part, answer them honestly. I reckoned it to be a welcome reprieve from the same idle chit-chat about sports, the weather, politics, movies, and what have you that usually accompanies a haircut. I would spare them the more ghastly and visceral details, of course, there being no need to make the situation uncomfortable. I would lay out the bare bones of the story in what would in time become a well-rehearsed spiel. I would answer questions as best I could and inject snippets of humour whenever possible to demonstrate that I had accepted the circumstance with levity and resolve. The vast majority, particularly the women, would express a heartwarming mix of sympathy and admiration for what I had endured, as if congratulating me on having such a positive outlook and jovial demeanour about the subject.

Occasionally the more talented and aware would comment on manners in which the incident had affected how my hair grows, how the follicles had been altered in this way or that, leading to an extreme cowlick or a variance in coarseness. Overall, they would work around the scar in such a way as to keep it more clandestine while helping to style my hair so as to account for the rebelliousness of the aforementioned cowlick. Professionals acutely aware of the importance of appearance to self-worth, they would proceed on the presumption, not incorrectly, that my scar caused some damage to my self-esteem.

By the time I arrived in Calgary from Vancouver, it had been a couple of decades of booze and drugs, women and restaurants, laughter and sorrow since the teenage days of insecurity in Nova Scotia. I was acutely aware of my scar but hardly gave it a moment's thought. My career and social life had begun to take off and I was able to define myself in my own terms. Recently separated from my wife and about to embark on a new culinary experience at a now renown izakaya, I felt empowered and unhindered. Goals were set and clear. Life seemed fecund with possibility and promise. Again, my hair was reaching a length that I felt suited me, a Samson-esque testimony to the strength I promoted from within.

Free from the criticism of an unkind and judgemental wife, I began to sport a goatee that would descend nearly to my chest. I was a talented and knowledgeable chef and a familiar and respected face in the metal scene. Single and happy, driven and jovially rambunctious, I had never felt more myself. I had worked hard to establish myself as a professional so I could represent myself physically without reproach. Sure, I may have looked like an '80s crime drama dirtbag dealer, but I brought *cuisine nouveau* and classic together with a global flourish. There was no longer any question of insecurity, of self-doubt.

I had practically achieved my desire to be free to express myself undaunted and unapologetically. Pride and passion had taken root and flourished, nurtured by the bounty of respect and admiration around me. That long-haired metal kid from rural Nova Scotia had found his footing and progressed toward a goal of being a freakshow metal chef of some esteem, a coif of power crowning him ostentatiously.

Previously detailed events had arrested the progress to those goals. A new scar was now in place as a reminder. Having just returned from the barbershop down on 11th Ave., five blocks away, I sit before my laptop and reflect on my freshly shaved mohawk. The slight breeze that permeated the warmth of early April sun caressed soothingly the exposed skin as I meandered pensively home moments before. Having had my head prepped for surgery over five years earlier, I have had ample time to grow out my hair. I, however, go through periods in which I have it shaved down on the sides, leaving length down the middle to drape nonchalantly over scarcely concealed scars. I often use fibre putty and gel to slick back my hair, the scars overtly displayed.

Erstwhile days of feeling insecure about the surgical hallmarks of traumas endured have been supplanted by extended periods of visual proclamation of survival. Those scars that streak precisely and dominate, jagged and insistent, across my scalp have become emblematic of my struggles and triumphs alike.

Over the past few years, as I've indicated, I would have my head shaved professionally as a silent declaration of tenacity and perseverance. The first shearing, however, was an amateur hack job. One night, having ignored medical advice, I had tied one on in the company of a close friend. Drunk and feeling rebellious, I made the decision and he offered to take up the clippers on my behalf, assuring me he had given dozens of mohawks through the years.

In short, I wanted *Taxi Driver* and got *Simple Jack*.

The result of his inebriated attempt was reminiscent of a bowl cut gone awry. Far removed from the empowering image of a scarred and triumphant survivor I had envisioned. I looked more like someone who had lost a bet. The situation was rectified forthwith upon awakening in the morning to a mirror that only seemed to mock my intentions. The only other time I would let a non-professional perform the task thereafter would be that same friend's two young children. Of course, I was again under the influence. It too would need repair by the hands of a trained barber.

Thereafter I'd have scheduled visits to the same barber every two weeks. Skilled hands wielding the clippers that reveal the extent of the scars deftly, so that at any time I could gaze at my reflection and cogitate leisurely on all that had come to pass. The emblematic nature with which I have imbued those scars gives me strength and pride in times of distress. Therein exists physical evidence of resilience, of a conquering will.

Perhaps there are some strangers in the street or at the bar that find them distracting, disturbing, or distasteful, but I couldn't give two drops of hot spit about that. The striving and struggling I have known are my own and how I perceive my scars, recognize them, and celebrate them is mine alone, requiring neither justification nor explanation. The scars mark me as more than a survivor; they brand me as more than a victim. They are a badge, a sigil, and a talisman.

Far from defining me, they stand for my capacity for self-definition.

15
THE MAZE OF IFS

There is another bottle of shiraz in my periphery as Beethoven fills my ears once again. I am alone. I have been alone for a fairly long time now. I have mostly grown accustomed to it and hardly give it a second thought. I have become disinterested in physical contact, in part out of fear that such an occurrence might trigger a glitch in the limbic system, and I'd respond inappropriately.

I don't date. I don't fuck. I don't spend a moment of my waking life intimately vulnerable with anyone. Besides a recent night, I have gone a year without so much as kissing a woman.

Obviously, my last relationship is a major factor.

Watching, helpless and angry, as the woman you love turns into a revenant of her former self is a devastating deterrent. Rattled and tattered from meth, a rainbow fading and tarnished. That itself might be enough to push a man into solitude and reclusion. Beneath that glaring, unpleasant truth of what she was going through was what I was enduring. I was not yet a year out of surgery when she and I began dating. As my brain still collapsed sometimes under the strain of mere existence, I found myself strolling hand in hand down her rabbit hole. While I needed nothing more than stability and calm, I was upended repeatedly by chaos, trauma, drama, and pain. This for nearly two years. Again and again, the revenant would appear, would thrust or creep itself into my life, and I would let it in. My fresh synaptic pathways not able to distinguish sour from sweet, I couldn't fully perceive the danger. Besides, I used to be able to help any I cared for, help them back to a life that was more familiar for them. Why should this be different?

I soon discovered that I no longer had all the tools for such a task. Furthermore, I couldn't properly wield the ones I had. The patience, the calm, the empathic yearning to understand and relieve the pain of a loved one seemed cumbersome and unbalanced. I was prone to confusion and anger, denial and intolerance. My emotional brain was by no means up to the challenge. Brutal fights and soul-crushing separations. Each time the spectre of the girl I knew, the woman I loved would return worn thinner than before and my brain would erupt like a fireworks warehouse with destructive misfires of impulsivity and altruism. Love and dopamine whispering sweet nothings under the gossamer canopy of encephalomalacia, I was blinded by the display and suffocating on the smoke.

For months I would get trapped in the inescapable maze of *ifs* my mind would create. I would imagine a life unfettered by such calamities as drugs and deceptions, loss and regret. If only I had not suffered that damn brain injury, I would chime in my head, how different it would have been. I would have had the clarity to see the answers, the emotional strength to hear the harsh and terrible truths without panic. Had my intellect not been hindered, and my cognizance not been impaired by boots and concrete, would I not have been able to provide her with all she needed? Had I not been so freshly out from under the surgeon's scalpel, would I have likely accepted her invitation to be inclusively together when she had first suggested it months earlier? I'm sure I would have. I had carried a flame, as they used to say, for years. Again, the gates to the maze of *ifs* creaks open. I no longer enter, the easiest solution to that maze being not to step inside. This I say as I again peer inside.

Len Roach

A mere month after my surgery I was invited to a friend's place, her place. She had explained a couple weekends earlier that she and her long-time boyfriend had split up for good. On account of his fentanyl addiction and subsequent unlawfulness, he was not only out of her basement apartment, but out of the province lest warrants catch up to him. In my mentally fragile state, I was oblivious to her undertones of interest. I explained that I was leaving romantic and sexual life behind. I was in no shape to handle the implications of anything of the sort. Later, she would tell me how I didn't notice her face drop as disappointment clasped at a tender place in her heart. I hadn't noticed and thus didn't give it a moment of thought when I agreed to go visit her in her basement apartment one night.

After having drinks upstairs with her friend and landlord of six years, we made our way down into the dimly lit apartment below. I had been to her place dozens of times in the past, drinking bourbon and smoking up while movies played, laughter filling the air. I felt comfortable there. It was familiar territory. The familiarity was soon peppered increasingly by vibrations of intent. Her use of language began to fill the air with innuendos and double *entendres*. Her movements and gesticulations punctuated her words as she made her desires more overt.

I, still in a post-traumatic stupor, was slow to catch on. My mind, at ease with having recognized the familiarity of my surroundings, was not prepared for these unexpected proceedings. Before I fully inferred what she was suggesting, or at about the same time, impulsivity took the reins and charged headlong into the instantaneous spontaneity of a yearning I had harboured for years. My prior proclamation of abstinence was unacceptable to her, so she felt to stage a convincing rebuttal. Indeed, she did so with great success.

The details of our encounter I have opted to spare you. Perhaps during editing or in some more lurid retelling, I shall parade my smut across the page like a dime-store Rimbaud. Perhaps one day I shall take up the mantle of Henry Miller and paint vast panoramas of fuckery and vice, but not here and not now. Of the deed itself I will only regale with two moments, the first being the moment my attending her needs was interrupted by a most audible whelp of pain as her fingernails buried into the tender, delicate flesh of a scalpel-drawn incision along my scalp. Pleasure was momentarily vanquished by bewildering pain and distress. The second moment was immediately after, when all the release and calm of post-orgasmic titillation seemed to soothe and clarify my mind. A stillness and serenity seemed to settle serendipitously between frontal and apex, between spine and sternum. I felt calmer, more self-aware than I had since I awoke drugged and shaven in a hospital bed over a month earlier. The dull, aching drone of head trauma abated for several moments of inner peace, leaving only the soft chortling of serotonin.

In short, I felt fantastic—not surprisingly, as the post-coital hum of pleasure was still reverberating through my body, as it would with anyone. I hadn't felt so good in weeks and said as much. She responded with something about her "magic pussy," a common tactic of diverting focus superficially onto herself that would be a vein running the length of our relationship. The pituitary gland having been spurred into action, I was flooded with oxytocin, endorphins, and vasopressin. Though this surge of hormonal sedation of pain and anxiety was dwindling slowly to a trickle, I was still in its embrace as she began speaking of her interest in me being her only lover. My lateral orbitofrontal cortex, which had been severely damaged in my teens and recently further affected, was just coming back to full readiness. That part of the brain shuts down to a degree during sex, limiting the anxiety and fear while inhibiting the faculties of decision-making, reasoning, and evaluation of situations. Damaged and somewhat subdued, it struggled with the prospect of pursuing a relationship with her. That I had already followed whim and fancy into actions I had sworn off a mere two weeks prior and the fact that immediately after she started talking of previous partners was not settling at all well. I did care for her and had for a long while.

The idea and the circumstances coalesced into the incalculable, the overwhelming. It was at this point I realized that I was nowhere near the state of mental acuity or emotional stability to take on such a venture. The fact that I was dumbfounded by the proposal itself was enough to validate my reluctance. So, when she asked, "What if I asked you to be my only?" I said, "I'd have to say no."

We proceeded with our late-night passions. Perhaps a drink or a smoke may have interrupted the sweat-glazed entanglement from time to time, but we did proceed. To be honest, this was to me not far removed from the tasks assigned while in therapy. I was somewhat detached and only heeded the call of performance itself. Solve the puzzle. The puzzle was pleasure. Do it as best you can. Focus on the task at hand. A robot feeling human joys and motivations, a joyous and motivated human processing cause and effect like a robot. The night continued until the early hours, dawn singing its hymnal of promise and light. The matter of our union, both physical and the other, seemed to have fallen by the wayside and recuperative life as I knew it would stumble onward, abated only by the trials and tribulations of severe head trauma.

After missing a therapy appointment a week or two later, I stopped answering when she called. Eventually, she took the hint and stopped calling. After my continuous reiteration of the state of my well-being, which needed to be my primary concern, all communication ended. Missing that appointment after hours of being drawn into her troubles over the phone until daybreak would be the point of severing ties.

I would go on without her. Intent on being uninvolved and focused on healing, I did not suspect or predict that I would be dating soon after. I had met a sexy Icelandic punk rock girl with a penchant for fun and drink. As far as the aforementioned, she too had moved on. The phone calls and text messages had ceased. We did not talk and lived our lives separated by our individual and mutually exclusive situations. My situation changed as it became obvious that

I was not prepared mentally to decipher the emotional components of a relationship. Trauma had left me far too needy and impatient. Limbic jitters and spasms painted abstract presumptions. It didn't end well, but it didn't end with lingering hostility. The girl from my previous fairy-tale delusion, however, had met a wolf. There was nothing there abstract or imagined, only cruel and abhorrent acts of abuse she suffered at the hands of drunk. Absolutes in shades unkind and destructive.

The stage is set. This lengthy preamble has given the necessary information to perhaps make the following more relevant. The next part is difficult. To be honest and truthful, I will need to delve deep into the folds of time and cerebrum. I am, however, drained and depleted, unable to advance farther in. For now, I must sleep, rest my weary mind and body. I wonder if I will dream as I once did of her smiling on a sunlit shore, the ocean breeze caressing her loose red hair soothingly. I wonder if I will dream at all.

A couple of wine-induced slumbers later, I ventured to address the matter anew. I will not get into too much detail, as it isn't my place to say. I will insist that you accept that the level of degradation and abuse she endured at the hands of the man she was with left her scarred and fragmented. It echoed through her, reverberating behind her eyes. The shame and pain led to anger and self-loathing. She was escaping moment by moment from memories, from the outrage through any means at hand. Cocaine, bourbon, and crystal meth flung open doors of instant gratification, the latter all smoke and mirror illusion of dopamine and insight. Before my eyes, she withered away. I knew how and why it began. I knew of her turmoil, the torture to which she had been subject. She came to me in pain, wanting nothing more than love, love she knew was there nestled beneath that canopy of encephalomalacia. It was entirely overwhelming, and I responded very poorly at times. Where one would expect me to be sensitive, I would be combative. Situations that called for tact, tenderness, and willingness to listen would be greeted with a desperate need to flee, shut down, or divert. Somewhere within, the spectre in my mind would watch in muted silence as I would erupt in a drunken rage at her inability to perceive the effects of her addiction. Of course, I see the irony now as I could see it then. I could also see clearly how differently our tale would have unfolded had I not suffered that brain injury. If I had not been effectively robbed of my capacity for understanding, not denied temporarily my trust in my own emotions, then it would have been different. If only I had been able to say "Yes" when she had asked the first time, how much better would things have been? The possibilities made me weep as I turned the same corner in that maze of *ifs* again and again, day after day, for months.

I blamed myself. Not only for my erratic behaviour or emotional outbursts, but those excesses of response also spurred into frenzy by misfires of a damaged brain. The fault, the guilt I felt did not stop at the shame and disgust after lashing out verbally and screaming unpleasant and cruel things until police knocked assertively at the door in the middle of the night. The guilt I felt was for my inability to be the man I had been a year before, when I was able to process and react with more decorum and care. I would wake the morning after a night of thorns ashamed of my response, my actions, and who I had become.

The drink didn't help. It threw fuel on my mind, which was already ablaze in frustration and confusion, reacting in volatile ways. Primarily, I was crestfallen to the point of angry defeat. That I was no longer able to help someone I cared for made it worse in many ways. From the beginning I would react irrationally to anything too dramatic, too intense. The night she spoke of what she endured I stepped into delirium. I made her stop telling me. I asked her to leave. I punched a hole in the wall and tried to lock myself in the bathroom. A sudden and pronounced breakdown possessed me as my mind lurched desperately away from what I was hearing.

Drunk and overwhelmed by the horrors flashing before my mind's eye, I only made her feel unsafe and concerned for my well-being. Later, she would tell me it broke her heart. Lament for who I had been led me to try to be a better person, a better companion to her. She still carried anger and pain at all that had happened by the other's hand, anger that would erupt after having too many drinks, needing to be released regardless of the target. Both she and I were by no means in a place to embrace each other without consequence. They say in case of loss of cabin pressure you must put on your own mask first. I wasn't doing that—strange, because I'd heard that said in therapy more than once in the previous weeks.

Her ability to bury and forget her trauma from abuse would falter with increased frequency. The same could be said of my ability to face our individual traumas simultaneously without a drink. The drink arrived more often than not sporting the tattered dream coat of an irrational mind. How we would squabble and scream, each trying to express the very thing we sought to suppress. Irritants and discomforts bloomed into orchards of fragrant disgust, love's tender proses were too often superseded by raging accusations, insults, and judgements. She blamed me for the abuse and the degradation by another's hand. On more than one occasion she would tell me if I hadn't rejected her previously, she never would have been in the situation, never would have got involved with the man that tortured her.

Overwhelmed by the possibility that I could be in part responsible, my mind spun out of control in hysterical overreactions. Later I would repay equivocally such baseless admonishments with heartless rebuttals of shame and mockery. Far from the nearest recollection of self, a man that looked and sounded like me spewed venom and disdain in a desperate attempt to distance himself from what only hurt and angered to hear.

The negativity that had at first only appeared at a frequency and potency common in any given relationship would become a resounding tone underscoring the opus. Resentment conquering sympathy as distrust vanquished affection; we would slowly disavow and distance ourselves. Originating as a chiming that sounded like misplaced notes only to decay into silence, the tone would change. Forgiveness would never fully be accepted as it was never properly given. This was true of both of us. Stockpiles of ammunition would build behind closed doors, before smiling eyes. Every slighting I perceived needed to be examined, re-examined, and understood. A brain in repair had no business trying to chart those waters, especially with a drink in my hand. I would dredge and delve into days gone by, reopening case after case. The din of negativity howling along, I needed to find a reason for it all. All the while I would attempt to ease her pain, ease her mind. Whether it be a bout of confusion, sorrow, or frustration, I would strive to right my course and assure her I was OK. It was just another bad brain day, no cause for alarm. Her sense of security notwithstanding, I needed to convince myself that I would be able to handle the relationship. After all, I had wanted it for years. I was, however, not able to fully grasp how my condition was contributing to the very negativity that assailed us.

On Boxing Day, we had a fight. We had just returned to her place from the hospital. We had spent the previous thirty-six hours at the Peter Lougheed Centre.

Christmas plans had been circumvented by the discovery that she had miscarried. An ectopic pregnancy caused not just her miscarriage but the rupture of one of her fallopian tubes. Being a contributor, I did not leave her side for two days except to work four hours and to get fresh air for thirty minutes while she slept after surgery. I slept for a total of three hours out of thirty-six. I was there for what she needed when she needed it, to the best of my ability. Gifts and snacks, company and attention, I did as I thought was proper. I was with her before and after she underwent the procedure to have what was our shared conception removed. I was by her side when she returned home, weakened and in pain. I held her hair as the bourbon and painkillers surged out. I helped her onto the bed when dizziness and fatigue sapped her of her strength. When she asked me to lend her my phone so she could get some drugs delivered, I advised against it. I was open to discussing the possibility and said so; I just wanted her to lie down first. I also flew off the handle and stormed out after she bellowed, "I don't need you to be my fuckin' dad right now!"

Quickly I gathered my things and expressed my outrage to be addressed with such impudence. Bourbon and exhaustion quelling rational thought, I fled to the nearest bar. I drank with strangers that had invited me to join them after a few minutes sitting alone in a country bar in the northeast while my girlfriend, healing from surgery, was doing lines in a house on a cul-de-sac somewhere in Falcon Ridge.

Forty dollars later, a cab dropped me home. Alone in my apartment, my fragile mind throttled by whiskey and draft, I succumbed to the Siren's song rumbling in the underscore. Everything negative and ill-conceived would be retrieved or created. Another flight-or-fight dilemma to which I had become prone had yet to reach its conclusion and the latter had taken the upper hand. An intoxicated and beleaguered limbic system was spastic and convoluted as fragments of truth and fantasy intertwined nonsensically.

When she answered her phone, I was already squawking a diatribe of disappointment and damnation. I had done so much, had been by her side, had been a beacon of love, attentiveness, and support. I gave of myself all I had to give to remain strong and composed, despite the anxiety and fear that enveloped me while I was within hospital walls. For this I was essentially told to mind my place, to fuck off. The drink convinced my ego that this was inexcusable, and I ended things. The underscoring tone had reached a crescendo of sorts, like a wave crashing hard.

For months I only knew the lack of her and regret. She would not speak to me. Having hurt her deeply, I found myself weeping, drinking, and wallowing in lament. I was denied the opportunity to make amends. The instability of mind echoing in my head, the calamity of my actions filled me anew with shame. My callousness shocked her. She could never have thought me to be so cold, so obstinate, and so apathetic. I couldn't either. I was forced to accept that I had cast aside all that I had wanted for so long, removed from my life she who had at one time been my greatest source of happiness, of joy. The painting I had started for her remained unfinished and would become a focal point of distraction and discovery as I waded my way through the mire of my regrets and the nature of my situation. I took to brush and bottle. The drink continued unabated as the canvas slowly filled with acrylics. I would send emails in lieu of texting, poetically composing my remorse. In the hours of staring blankly as memories formed behind my bloodshot eyes, somewhere between lachrymose displays and temporal scars, her face would appear, her eyes a vivacious blue shimmer. Unable to find the mental agility to avoid or deflect the barrage of emotions, I sank deep beneath the waves. I remained submerged for days on end, perhaps weeks. The canvas would be testament to my devotion. If ever we were to reunite, she would have proof that she had never strayed far from my thoughts. As it took shape, so did my mind. The sorrow had begun to subside and again I could find peace and contentment. Confidence and fortitude having returned, I reached out again.

It's hard to stay focused. The delirium and derangement of those months flicker in and out of distorted memory with little regard for chronology. She and I would talk and text again with increasing frequency. She respected my request not to hear of her boyfriend and their relationship. There was much else to discuss anyway. For example, she had been locked out of her place for not paying rent. Citing complications with federal employment insurance, she insisted that she was being fucked over by her long-time friend and his mother. They were renting the place to her, and she'd known them for years. It wasn't her fault. It never was. When she was finally able to get Calgary Police to accompany her to retrieve her plethora of belongings, she still hadn't secured a place to live. I offered to store this and that, my sympathy and adoration having been reignited by weeks of contact and her harrowing tale of mistreatment, bad luck, and betrayal. I saw it as a chance to, at minimum, make up for earlier misdeeds. The months of introspection, exercise, and art had reset the balance drinking had thrown off. My mind needed to test its progress, its resolve. I had to prove to myself that I was well on the mend and able to rein in irrational, explosive responses. It should be a foregone conclusion that I overestimated my ability for patience and perseverance.

In my defence, her situation had changed drastically. She, too, had changed. The vivaciousness and vitality seemed artificial. A forced evanescence had draped itself over something unfamiliar like a veil. I would sidestep the questions as they cropped up in my mind, not wanting to open doors that in the past had only released confusion, panic, and fear. I knew something had changed but couldn't muster the courage or confidence to consider what it could be. I was so happy to have her back in my life: an opportunity to edit, rewrite, and improve the past. Whatever the change was, whatever it was that had cast this notable shadow, mattered not. I was sure-footed, strong in mind and spirit. I could handle and solve any problem.

I overestimated indeed.

They say love is blind. They say love conquers all. They say love is a many-splendoured thing. All that could very well be true, but I can attest with certainty that love is one of the great disinhibitors of all time. The reward and risk factors are thrown into a disproportionate tailspin. Tidal bores of dopamine surging with ferocious regularity fill one's head with such pleasant delusions and phantasms, producing a warmth from within that is like no other, which inspires and elevates, operates more delicately with the same tools addiction destroys. The frontal cerebral cortex is the playground, the flower-strewn meadow in which love flourishes gracefully. It is also the abattoir, the slaughterhouse killing floor where crystal meth performs its macabre theatre. The chemicals she had been injecting disturbed the processes of her mesolimbic pathway. No longer capable of adequately producing or even receiving dopamine naturally, she could not allow the love I had for her to penetrate her addiction. Withdrawal meant sorrow, stress, and traumatic recollection that she could not stave off. In and out of my life she would stumble and fall. The pipe in time would be replaced with syringes; the love would be replaced by disdain. I would return to alcohol to numb the pain. It muffled the desperate, wailing thoughts in my traumatized brain. It blurred the image of my beautiful friend, my pretty one, as she slowly disintegrated. The memory of her naked before a mirror, gouging purposefully at invisible bugs beneath her skin until a dozen miniscule rivulets of blood marred her pale arms and neck still breaks me. All her pain and delusional desperation ensnared me, compelling me to seek woeful refuge of my own.

My drinking only proved to retrograde any progress toward mending my damaged brain; impulsivity issues I had always known were now explosive. I became destructive and, on one occasion, violent, throwing her to the floor. I would revert to the irrational and often cruel responses that seemed to somehow circumvent my faulty rational centres all together. The comfort and support I had promised with sincerity and purest intention had been replaced with what she called hatred. I believe a preternatural instinct for survival had caught the wave of boozing and rode it hard up from a place deep and reptilian within. Striking out again and again, I would drive her from my domain once and for all. Her lies and manipulations, her drug-fueled egotism, and her thieving dirtbag friends all had to be exiled. My attempts to save her from drowning had pulled my head beneath the waves too often and long enough.

It was hard to admit defeat, hard to admit I had failed her. It was not how I wanted it, but knew it was how it must be. I no longer had the resilience to take on so many demons at once. The depth of thought and emotional control I had painstakingly redeveloped for two decades since my first craniotomy, though far from perfect, were now again significantly impaired. I could barely help myself. I couldn't help her. Crystal meth may have taken away the woman I loved and replaced her with a tragic counterfeit, but those bastards that put me in the hospital took away any chance I had of re-animating her. This I shall never forgive.

She hasn't been a part of my life for than a couple years now. I have no idea where she is. I don't even know if she is alive or dead, and can never know. To find out would only bring chaos and pain.

She was here and now she is not.

I loved her and I wish this wasn't so.

16

CHINOOKS: A TROUBLING REPRIEVE

My first winter in Calgary was brutal. It was cold and bombarded with storms aplenty. No slouch when came to winter storms on account of my upbringing on the Northumberland Straight in Nova Scotia across the water from PEI, I was still at a disadvantage in terms of weather after so many years spent in Vancouver. The drop in temperature and seemingly endless snowfall were familiar enough that I was able to quickly adjust, reverting to my rural self and confronting the winter armoured in layers of preparation. It hadn't been so long since I was last at the mercy of Atlantic storms bottlenecking their way up Pugwash River. The marked difference was the phenomenon known as a Chinook.

Those sporadic and appreciated days of sudden warmth and calm that settle over southern Alberta, enveloping it in a life briefly more pleasant, more easily navigated, are born of Chinook winds—dry, gusting winds rolling down from the Rockies elevating temperatures by double digits and devouring the drab grey of an urban setting engulfed in snow and squall. For the first few years of my time in Calgary, I greeted the Chinook winds with gratitude. As much as I had acclimatized relatively quickly to the reality of winters here,

Skull Fragments

I still very much longed for the mild stupor of West-Coast rainy seasons from time to time. Chinooks brought the warmth without the stone-grey sky fecund of rain. I, like most, enjoyed these "snow-eating" winds as a reprieve, though a brief one, from the hassles of winter, and waited countless frigid hours in the interim between.

Well enough over a year after awakening in the hospital after an emergency craniotomy I was working at a popular and acclaimed Italian restaurant on Eighth. It was near enough to my apartment that I was able to walk there in about fifteen minutes in rain or snow. One night, the snow was falling heavy and thick, coating the city in a formidable layer of cold, white hindrance. I was well enough aware that I would require more time to reach my destination the following morning and so made necessary preparations. I awoke early with a mild headache, but thought nothing of it. I likely just needed to hydrate and get some grub into my guts. As the morning advanced, the sun rose high on the horizon. It was brighter and more assertive than on previous days, as though sanctifying the return of those westerly winds from the mountains, revealing a world of drifted snow and barren sidewalks. My walk to work would be of no ordeal, save the growing pressure behind my eyes. I had never been adversely affected by the benevolent shift brought forth by Chinooks, as many are. I had heard of migraines and insomnia as side effects of the dramatic shift but had not experienced it in the first few winters. The first winter after my surgery would be different as I would discover as I lumbered toward my job nearby.

The mild weather permitted me to wear a ball cap, which I had pulled down purposefully around my brow to shield me from the sunlight, which was more malicious and discomforting than I had ever known. Aviators and the brim of my hat performed adequately in the assigned task of protecting newly sensitive retinas from solar assault. So it was that I trudged alone in notable discomfort, confident that the pain behind my eyes would eventually abate. Perhaps it was as much denial as disbelief that lessened my concern for the predicament, though there was, as there understandably can be, the notion that it could involve my brain injury. That was my thought as I walked around the corner of a sandwich shop and habitually removed my sunglasses as I would on any other day. My eyes were greeted by the sun reflecting on the snow-covered parking lot like shards of luminescent glass. Pain shot through my ocular cavity and into my brain as my knees buckled beneath me. Catching myself against the wall, I yelped nearly inaudibly and replaced my sunglasses before unlocking the restaurant and starting my shift.

The calamitous change in barometric pressure would spike into my ocular cavity, penetrating my skull as light from the fluorescent bulbs overhead was scarcely muted by the tinted glass of my sunglasses still nestled on my face. This is how I would start my day, squinting to near blindness and fumbling around in great, bewildering discomfort. I continued the processes of opening the kitchen for service as if it were any other day. I was greatly impeded, and it showed. I was slower and far less jovial than normal. Wincing and muttering condemnations under the low vibrato of the kitchen fan, I persevered. My situation was obviously far from ideal and clear to all who were present. I wasn't prone to kowtowing to weakness or letting a physical ailment defeat me. It was pride, of course. I took pride in having overcome my brain injury and was unwilling to let myself be downed by a consequential trifle like Chinook sensitivity. I would press on until the chef got in. He commended me on my fortitude for having stayed so long, for having come in at all. He did so as he ushered me out the door to return home. I was damn near an invalid as I arrived home. The two hours at work I spent suffering was not an act of bravado but an act of denial. I couldn't accept the idea that I could be prone to Chinook migraines—to do so would require my considering the ramifications of it happening every fucking time. I ruminated on the dreadful anxiety of it every time the forecast called for it.

I had another occurrence recently, but at a different restaurant this time. I wasn't greeted in the morning with an early strumming of internal discord. I was already well lodged into my daily routine at work when it happened. I was lighting the fire and stocking my station as I would on any another day, the frivolity and quirkiness I was exuding indicative of my good spirits. Within a few brief minutes, I was again donning dark glasses and recoiling from bright lights. A momentary venture outside for fresh air left me slumped on a milk crate in the shadows, wincing visibly as tears flooded my eyes. The pain, the strain, and the anxious foreboding had shuttered my tearful, reddened eyes as again I felt the weight of ill possibilities pile on. Though it had been years since that first devastating bout and the intermediate ones had been subjectively mild, I was still at the mercy of a panic and agitation that could only worsen my condition if I were to let it take hold. Once again it was my chef that intervened. How could he not? My response to his asking how I was doing was to describe the worst as being like someone was slowly driving their thumbs behind my eyes and the best like a steady drumming, like impatient fingertips on a desk. He had never seen anything like it; the drastic change I underwent was from happily focused and jovial to leaning near motionless sipping chamomile tea in sunglasses. I was relieved of my obligation to work and allowed to slink home to submerge myself in total brain rest.

While enveloped in as much darkness and silence as I could muster up, I reminded myself of the potential that if ever these frequent and pervasive Chinook winds became prone to assail me then I would need to leave. The sensitivity I feel in and for my brain and its legacy of torment and struggle would demand of me nothing less than relocation. Thus far there has been no need to commence such preparations, but, should the time come, I would walk away from any and all. The pain, extreme as it is, can only do lasting harm and the anxiety it wields like an ax most certainly will. Those warm days do whisper memories and longing for spring like seductive zephyrs that croon Demeter choruses amid the dead of winter. Let not too often trauma lurk in wings, waiting to scream.

17
MOSH PITS AND NEUROLOGY

I told this story to my friend just today while we chomped down burgers of the messy and delicious variety at a local franchise bar. It was a lunch of brevity and reconnection after months of limited contact due to COVID restrictions, so there was some catching up to do. It also marked the first time we could have a proper face-to-face conversation since my second brain surgery. He had some questions.

He was flying back to Vancouver in a few hours, and we had not been able to meet in a less time-sensitive moment than just after his twelve o'clock checkout from a downtown hotel, a meagre few hours before his departure. I didn't want to see him off with the usual, well rehearsed spiel. I wanted to share something more lighthearted to leave a less clinical tone resounding.

As should be obvious and thus not requiring extrapolation, I had undergone extensive therapy to help me recuperate from a significant brain injury. A brief summary is months of vocational, physiological, occupational, and psychological therapy followed by hours of testing my cognitive functions. Hence the questions and concern he had. The testing went exceedingly well considering the extent of my injuries. All this led ultimately to a sit-down meeting in an expansive and expensive office that belonged a neuropsychologist.

In his due diligence he went through the rigmarole of reviewing my file: testing, scores, assessments, and the like. He was the man to make the call for me to return to normal life as an employed taxpayer. My efforts and tenacity coupled with results of my rigorous testing had guided him to the obvious conclusion that I was ready to return to life as I knew it. Well, sort of. There were still a few T's and I's that required their respective crossing and dotting.

In preparing me for my return to life approximately as I had known it before the surgery and before the therapy, it was necessary to discuss certain limitations I had acquired throughout my ordeal. There was the discussion of a return-to-work plan, which had already been begun. He also brought up recreational interests. The doctor, seated comfortably behind his desk, asked whether, prior to my assault and subsequent injuries, I had been involved in any sports. He was particularly interested in my involvement in contact sports like MMA, boxing, hockey, and the like. I told him that I was not athletic.

He rephrased the question for certainty's sake, citing the importance that I avoid any activity that had a high chance of exasperating my condition or worse. I reiterated that I did not play any sports in my free time, particular not extreme sports or the contract sports he had mentioned. I did, however, add that the closest thing to an extreme sport I did participate in was mosh pits. He looked at me quizzically from across the dark wood of his fastidiously maintained desk and asked with a gentle curiosity "What's a mosh pit?"

It was apparent that he had never heard of moshing at all. This I found surprising as it is relatively common to see it in some form or other in pop culture. References in movies and television being unfamiliar to him, I proceeded to explain what a mosh pit was to this curious but unaware neuropsychologist. The curious and congenial expression of general interest on his face slowly changed as I began to explain the ritual of moshing and mosh pits. As though witnessing a frame-per-second transformation, disbelief, bafflement, and concern shaped his visage into one of perplexed awe. Flashes of what could best be called outrage and disgust briefly sparked in his eyes as he stared, enraptured and stunned, at me, absorbing the description of events that constitute a mosh pit.

It was not long into my regaling him that he interrupted with questions. The doctor's disbelief and astonishment needed to be validated by the facts.

"You all actually . . . ?"

"Then you slam into each other?"

"You do this for how long?"

"How often?"

His quick-fire inquiries to get confirmation that he had heard me correctly were followed by a pause of no more than two seconds in which the befuddlement, disbelief, and outrage coalesced into an expression of stern and informed concern.

"No. No. No," he said, his head shaking from side to side as he leaned back in his chair. "No one, no."

The shock of what he'd heard had robbed him of his coherency for a moment.

"No one should be doing that. Ever!"

His words and breath having returned, the doctor exclaimed with absolute certainty that the purposeful jostling of the brain through moshing alone was reckless and not advised but coupled with randomly colliding into one another it was beyond that. This was clearly an affront to all he'd studied, knew and practised. Moshing was something he adamantly wasn't prepared to hear about.

"No one should be doing this, especially you and especially now," he concluded, engulfed in conviction and knowledge.

The timbre and tone denoted the seriousness of his stake.

The rapid shifts in expression and overall bewilderment still make me laugh.

18

SLEEPLESS ENCEPHALIC

Somewhere along the line there must have been a shift, an upwardly graded shift. For now, though, the room was silent, in lieu of my usual shiraz, I was drinking a Ripasso. However, that digression was grossly premature and likely utterly irrelevant save for the slight divergence from the usual.

It was forty-five minutes past midnight on a Thursday night in Calgary. January the 13th. Though my body was weary and worn from a night in the kitchen my mind was not. I suppose that's the meat of it. Nothing, in particular, was happening. Nothing, in particular, had. Yet my mind was darting within its cage, not content to skulk about forlorn through the battered creases and folds of an impaired brain.

I tried to control my thoughts, my mind. I tried to calm it. I tried to wait it out. It's not that I didn't want my mind to be exuberantly effervescent with questions and insights alike. In fact, I rather enjoy those near-blinding moments of full frontal synaptic enthusiasm when appropriate. The thing is I was just so fucking tired. My mind like a truffle pig of the existential foraging, I was unable to relax. I have enjoyed many a sun-flattered day in spring when such lively thinking revealed deeper splendour around me. However, when that same rambunctious deviant scamp opts for a nocturnal cortical exploration, it finds not the splendour within. To be honest, it doesn't make a lick of sense.

I lay there awake. I giggled to myself as my subconscious flung my mental focus about, willy-nilly, absurdly humorous to abjectly devastating and back. My mind's eye rivetted to a pendulum in a whirlwind of memories, fantasies, fears, and the simply fucking ridiculous. Thoughts on the feelings I experienced and the feelings I had about those thoughts haven't time enough to crystallize into anything identifiable before another spin about the skull distracted and deteriorated them. There was no shutting it off. The barrage of unexpected gems and unsolicited garbage was unyielding.

I tossed and turned in response. It was as though my body was tethered to the unhinged gyroscope my mind had become. Laughter and tears welled up from their respective sources in a cerebral tango that felt like a hatefuck. The one constant was a voice that insists in a calm monotonous droning. It hums, perpetually permeating throughout the cortical cavalcade of convoluted cacophony. The random assailants of past, present and peculiar rise and fall through it's axis like waves. It tells me to write.

Now that I've done that, I hope it is sated. I hope that the next time the absurdist philosopher child that resides behind the obligation for normalcy doesn't bolt toward the surface at an inopportune time, as has been the case in the past. I hope that my mind chases its cerebral gophers on a sedating Spring morning. I hope this primarily because I'm fucking tired and want to sleep.

19

DE BERGERAC OF THE MIND

The first time I kissed a girl was shortly after my fall from the roof of Pugwash District High School. It was around the corner of the front of the building on a warm autumn's day.

As it turned out my accident had caused her great concern, as she had been harbouring interest in me for days prior and wished to be my girlfriend. This was my first kiss with tongue and the primary step toward more adult interactions. After we had embraced and kissed, she explained that I must open my mouth more. Without a second thought I explained that I was incapable of opening my mouth beyond what I had as a result of the surgery I had undergone to repair the compound fracture of my eye orbit. I detailed how the surgeon had had to peel the muscle tissue from the bone just above my right mandible to facilitate the rolling down of the flesh of my forehead enough to attend to the severely damaged skull beneath. The cliche awkwardness of a first French kiss was magnified by my physical limitations having been brought to light, and more so by my ghastly and vivid explanation. This would not be the last time that an aspect of my cranial trauma would make an appearance in relationships, but when compared to the future to come it was by far the slightest inconvenience.

At this point it's prudent to iterate that I am very much single—more precisely, to reiterate that I do not currently date nor do I seek out one-night romps in the hay. With the exception of very rare occasions of booze- and drug-induced inhibition, I have been without a partner since well enough before the pandemic—long enough to make it feel like a different life, an alternate reality. Those few that are near me have accepted my status as single for the indefinite future, though some do not understand why. To most in my life I was perceived as an attractive, intelligent, funny, and thoughtful man—traits that are presumably desirable, but it's the undesirable traits that curtail my appeal.

When a friend came by to visit after our having not seen each other for nearly two years, due to the Coronavirus pandemic, he addressed his amazement that I was still alone. He was surprised that there was not a woman beside me that exuded the same qualities that so many find endearing in me.

Another close friend, having seen beyond my ruse, often expresses his hope that I find someone to share my life with. I've made my loneliness more known to him, albeit in snippets. How can I explain the true reasons, the rationalization of my opting for a life alone, despite the evident loneliness and yearning? I can barely come to grips with it myself at times. Often, I just repeat silently to myself that some are meant to be alone, for better or worse. I tell myself it's better this way. Often, I tell myself that no one needs this in their life, my charm, wit, and "classic good looks" notwithstanding.

Obviously, that one ex-girlfriend and our tumultuous relationship is a factor in my single life. I've touched on it enough already that I do not believe much more can be or needs to be added, save the admonishment that my instability did in no way facilitate an air of comfort and security even if she had made valid efforts to cease her descent down the rabbit hole into which she was to disappear.

Mood swings and overreactions, only exasperated by the drink, would continuously cause her post-traumatic impulses to rear up. Though my fluctuations of mood and mindset were at their worst in those early days of recovery from my second encephalitic injury, they have been a reccurring aspect of my life since my teenage years. To this day they persist, though fortunately to a degree I find relatively manageable provided I take ample stock and precautions.

I doubt the relevance of my teenage relationships. In regard to my brain damage those early romances are primarily inconsequencial. Youthful trysts and "puppy love" of any adolescent or young adult are wrought with confusion and befuddlement as unfamiliar waterways open and strange new terrains of emotions and hormones are suddenly found underfoot and abounding in all directions. Furthermore, the limitations of time spent together at such an age would have excluded certain experiences. I was not living with my girlfriends at fourteen, fifteen, or seventeen years of age. I would not share my space with a significant other for years. As a teenager, I was able to slink away into isolation if my moods and emotions became overbearing and uncontrolled. What times I couldn't were likely no different than those of any other young man being tossed about by the challenges and conundrums of adulthood's hormonal advancement. Similarly, I imagine those few young women of my high school dating history were likely unfamiliar with their own hitherto unknown waters and hadn't a basis from which to establish normalcy. I will move on from those distant and nearly forgotten years and try to sink my teeth into the meat of it all.

A few days ago, I was talking to my father about what I was like after my first accident. He told me about how he and my mother were never sure who would be coming home from school on any given day, who would be waking up any given morning. Such were the dramatic extremes in my mood and personality shifts—a common latent effect of damage to the orbital frontal cortex, though they didn't know that at the time. Common, too, is that very sentiment of not knowing what version of me will be in attendance at any given time. "I never know who I'm getting in the morning" has been a common-enough statement made by the women with whom I have shared my bed extensively. More often than not I would be at a loss to explain why I was acting or feeling so different. Perhaps it would be a bout of depression that would lull me into melancholy and indifference, so I would see no point in attempting to clarify or explain the situation. Perhaps it would be a more frustrated and bewildered version of myself that had manifested. I would simply be lacking the patience to delve into my troubles. Whatever the case might be, I would find myself not able to articulate properly the nature of my mental state.

Prior to the second craniotomy and the knowledge I gleaned through months of therapy, I hadn't any verified information to offer. I could only express my unsubstantiated believe that I had suffered a severe brain injury in my youth, and it was somehow still affecting me. Unable to elaborate in response to any follow-up questions due to lack of information, I was at a disadvantage, and left feeling *less than*.

I would often feel, early in a relationship, that my explanation devoid of details was viewed with suspicion and disbelief. After all, are not most brain-injured people depicted as severely challenged? I was employed and mostly self-reliant. Beyond that there would also be the comfort of deniability. There would, one can imagine, be a significant challenge to accept that someone for whom you had just begun to develop feelings could be potentially fighting an unseen battle of which they themselves understand so little.

There were relationships that I have had that did not require me to divulge many, if any, details, as they were flings of no substance beyond the physical. Conversely there were others that required full disclosure to the best of my ability, the bare bones of which I would lay out early enough. I'd show my scar and tell the tale of my fall. I would provide surface glimpses of facts of the accident from the outset of the relationship as a precursor to any future issues that might arise—and arise they normally would. A charming, positive man would hold the woman he loved close to him, crooning sensual reassurance and admiration as they drifted off to a soothing slumber. A darkened and dreary man would lie awake beside a confused and concerned beauty—she unable to understand, he unable to explain. I would know something was wrong and strongly suspected the cause, but I never fully knew the extent. After years of living that way, I just thought this was how I was. I felt shame and embarrassment. I felt deeply regretful that I was not able to provide a significant-enough explanation to appease or comfort for the times when loving eyes would look at me with helplessness, swimming in pools of concern. Or worse, when I would be asked if it was something they'd done. When your only response to the statement "I never know who I am waking up to" is "Me either," and you watch her face drop or hear her voice tremble ever so slightly, something inside resigns just a little. This is all through no fault of my own, beyond my control and understanding. An air of crestfallen disappointment permeates the room. A suppressed sigh interrupts the serenade, and none is, for a time, soothed. I would strive to clamour up out of the darkness in hopes of alleviating her of any woe begotten from her proximity to my own. Success in such an endeavour would vary, but often tenderness and my desire to be more would prevail over time.

Not all interactions are as sweet and reassuring as that. When the circumstances that lead to my discussing my brain trauma manifest on the tail end of recklessness or irresponsibility, the exchange can become argumentative and combative. A lost job or frivolous bout of spending can lead to stress and strain on any relationship, any marriage. In the moment, in the heated moment of an impassioned argument, one person can find themselves struggling to explain themselves and another can find themselves lashing out irrationally. An argument with my ex-wife about a recent job lose resulted in my attempt to explain my trouble considering consequences. I explained it was a possible result of my brain injury. That was met with venomous, maligned admonishment. Words that cut through my thin armour of regretful honesty, of open vulnerability. Having offered up my weakness, for which I felt shame, as an explanation that I had hoped would garner a semblance of support, I would be levelled and debased. The embarrassment I felt would be replaced by sadness which quickly turned to anger. The other person's audacity to mock me for something I cannot properly control for lack of knowledge was unacceptable. I would also lash out with cruelty of word. Feeling simultaneously exposed and trapped, my already overburdened emotional brain regressed to animal instinct and fight or flight were all that I knew. Loudly and unkindly, I would unload a torrent of judgement and insult as I sprinted to the door in an attempt to escape the confines in an extradition of self that would necessitate physically moving her from in front of the door. The pain of her words and the anger at her refusal to attempt understanding would override all other thoughts. Make haste and distance lest further faculties and better judgement succumb to the fires engulfing a beleaboured brain.

Perhaps it was best to keep it all to myself. It's not like I had received any therapy or even a comprehensive follow-up after the successful reconstruction of my skull, so how the hell could I have known?

Maybe I was simply a bit of an ass at times. Ill-informed and lacking in inhibition, perhaps I was doing nothing more than staggering through variant spontaneity. Being as familiar as any to the nature of my mood shifts and emotional instability, I was often less certain which version was interpreting events. Was I using that accident as an excuse? Was it really a factor or just a convenient means to justify capriciousness? Going to the walk-in clinic and asking for help only got me prescribed the pharmaceutical soup du jour. Trying to explain only brought more questions I could not answer. I wouldn't bring the matter up too often after that argument. I would just try in my whimsical and heartfelt way to be better.

Despite my attempts at more responsible behaviour, I fell short.

The ex-wife had witnessed a lot with me.

The times when my mood would sink into darkness. She had witnessed my seizures when I couldn't awaken from a dream. Though she was very much taken aback, she stayed with me and made me feel cared for.

It is through that relationship with my then-wife that I began to understand a sense of the magnitude of dealing with me, an undiagnosed head trauma survivor that only suspects his own predicament for lack of information. That could not have been easy. I do not doubt that my instability and outburst did erode the compassion she had. And for this I hold no ill will. She could not have known what I could not tell her in my ignorance of the dysfunction that was at play behind my eyes.

With the second brain injury, nearly two years after the wife left, I found myself in different hands. More than two decades had passed since my first and not only was there more information available, but I had access to it. Through the months of therapy, I gained not just knowledge but confirmation of what I had always suspected. The tumultuous history of mood swings, personality shifts, and general emotional disarray had been explained to a great extent. The tools and procedures for dealing with them had been provided. Despite the concerns and challenges, I was confident that I would not only survive but exceed and overcome my traumatic predicament. I was now in possession of pieces to the puzzle I didn't even know had been missing. Questions I had harboured for so many years were finally being answered. I was, despite the obvious challenges, in a better place to cope than I previously had been. Bolstered by knowledge and the team of professionals that provided it, I was eager to get to life as I had known it. My many therapists were appreciative of my enthusiasm and sought to help me any way they could. However, they would insist on my being cognizant of my limitations.

My return-to-work plan limited me to part-time work, no more than twenty hours a week. This so I would not be overwhelmed, overstimulated, or burnt out. After I had brought up the idea of again entering the dating world as a self-deprecating joke, one of my therapists (I believe my psychologist) insisted that I wait. She shared her concern that dating might prove taxing on my emotional brain. The areas that govern that kind of thing were damaged and my established predisposition toward excessive altruism was the foundation of her hesitation to encourage me. I took her advice to heart and swore off any such involvement. I agreed with her compassionate and logical belief that a relationship of a romantic sort would take too much time away from my brain. I needed to heal and realign. I couldn't allow such a distraction when there was such important work to do. This would be the thinking that led me to turn down one that I cared for deeply, one about whom I still wonder *what if?*

I would remain primarily focused on the work of healing and not much more. Twenty hours a week were devoted to my job and the rest were for me to heal and acclimatize to my new reality. No time for the pretty ladies.

Then I met someone. An enticing and spirited punk rock chick. Her cheekiness and playful irreverence paired nicely with my encephalitic spontaneity and boyish charm. We enjoyed each other's time immensely. Food and drink, laughter and lust. Frivolity abounded for the brief time we were in each other's lives. I was rapidly growing attached to and enamoured with her. Then one day she informed me that she wasn't in town. I thought we had tentative plans to spend the day together, but she told me she'd left for a British Columbia photo shoot.

I responded irrationally.

My brain was not yet accustomed to dealing with disappointment and I had a tantrum of sorts. She, rightfully and justly explained that she could go where and when she pleased. Though this was obviously true, I was still irrationally upset by her not at least letting me know. So it was that my brain misfired a few synapses and I felt wronged enough to pick a fight.

She had no interest in or time for such nonsense.

We had not been together long, not that that would justify my reaction had we been. She ended the conversation in frustration at my presumptuousness, having better things to do than validate my behaviour in any way. My befuddled and battered paleomammalian cortex hit the scene in a frenzy. I should have heeded my therapist's advice perhaps longer as I would respond disproportionately to what was merely the illusion of being slighted. After quickly deleting and blocking all means of communication with a woman that I found utterly delightful in every way, I settled into the drink again.

For two days I tried to convince myself I was right, that I had been treated with disregard. And after two days of deluding myself into believing such lies, my rational brain took the reins and my better self could be heard repeating in the darkness within: "What the fuck did you do that for?"

I had made a terrible mistake.

Unfairly, unjustifiably, I had shunned a sexy, smart, fun, and vibrant soul. I had walked away from someone who was effortlessly making me happy, all because I couldn't properly process emotional responses. What new, cruel torment was this that had befallen me? The realization of what I had done caused me to cringe, to suffer a gut punch of consequences and guilt. I had hurt myself with such reckless disregard. Moreover, I had hurt her. Her blocked text messages would tell me as much. I had made her feel disposable, or at least she thought that was my intent. My attempt to mend went as well as one might imagine. I had set a flame to trust and confidence, so even my assertion that my behaviour was a direct result of my brain damage would ring too much like a justification, an excuse, to me. I had thrust reluctance and hesitation onto her, had provided reason enough for her to say goodbye. I felt it best not to press the matter. Enough was happening in her life, an ample supply of struggles and bullshit alike. It was best she didn't have to deal with me as well. I could only explain my actions through a sort of depersonalized perspective, but couldn't excuse them. Nor could I be certain that I wouldn't have a similar occurrence in the future. Months later I would hear that she had been missing me, but by then, I was already lost in the spiral of another, on the precipice of someone's rabbit hole.

Prior to that misstep into monumental catastrophe that would engulf years of my life, I would explore the nature of my emotional instability for weeks after parting ways with that delightful punk woman. I spent the interim between my brief yet delightfully romantic involvement with an Icelandic spitfire and what was to follow focusing as much time and energy on my recovery as possible. I had accepted that I could not change the mistakes I had made, couldn't erase the consequences of my delusional reaction. I had only to try to improve. That first abundant helping of limbic malfunction left an aftertaste of regret and disappointment. I chastised myself for my arrogance, for convincing myself that I was fully capable of maintaining a relationship so freshly out from beneath the surgeon's blade. I'd wanted so badly to feel as though life had begun to resume a degree of normalcy that I'd cast aside reasonable doubt, which is not entirely a bad thing. That someone else was affected by my cerebral gambit was the problem. My tenacity when pushing myself beyond the minimum requirement was crucial and often applauded during most aspects of my recovery. This was one glaring example where my striving to reach beyond expectations and accepted limitations was a misstep. Not only was the resulting disappointment and heartache shared with a blameless and alluring young woman, but it planted the seed that was yet to germinate. The seed would sprout quickly into feelings of negative self-worth, of doubt in my ability to maintain stability. Would my inability to navigate emotions, mine and others, be the new hallmark? Those issues that had haunted me for years seemed to have amplified and I feared an irreversible new reality. If I were to remain so turbulent, so inconstant, it would be best to spare any future woman, right?

Before I knew it, I had again allowed my spontaneity and ignorance of risk lead me by the hand into another relationship. This next on-and-off cyclone of fuckery and pain lasted a couple of years. My brain, still in disrepair, was ill equipped for the myriad experiences that assailed and disrupted my recovery and daily life. The trauma, drugs, disillusionment, and general disarray have already been splashed on the page. I need not run my fingers through their viscosity again and I only mention them at all to make clear the uncertain shape those experiences left me in thereafter.

At that time, I was rocking the pans at a highly regarded pizza place in the Beltline neighbourhood of Calgary. I spent much of my downtime at work flirting playfully with one server or another in a mutually indulgent game of double entendre and innuendos with beautiful and charming young women that would never manifest into anything beyond mere flirtation. In hindsight, I believe there was a possible interest for more, but I would always sidestep it. I'd delve into my work or flash-bomb a self-deprecating joke to circumvent the inherent awkwardness of my deeply held belief that I was far too damaged from the previous months of turmoil. My lips would curl in a boyish smirk, I would break eye contact, and disappear the moment I sensed even a faint air of romantic interest. The aromas of attraction would fill my mind with what I could only assume were impossibilities. Shrinking away from the desire and attention, I would superimpose memories of pain and confusion to hoodwink such fanciful delusions. Not only did I have so little to offer, but what I did have had proven to be unstable too frequently. Though before me would stand a young woman, seemingly slightly enamoured and piquing my interests nicely, I could only consider her to be undeserving of the unpredictability and struggles to which I was heir. She could obviously do better. Besides, it would be wise to avoid such interactions at work. Those two notions were easily accepted as facts. I had made the decision to remain single, to forgo the obstacles of self-reflection that would come in tandem with anything akin to a romantic relationship. However, I must confess that one of the women I worked with touched me deeply. I harbour a smattering of regret regarding that, yet it remains somehow irrelevant.

Eventually, a very popular social media platform would soon have me second-guessing my choice to remain alone. It would start with riffing sarcastic and insightful, sensational, and facetious on-comment threads. The dialogue a stunning woman and I established became equal parts comedic, intelligent, and titillating. Before long we were messaging each other late into the night. All the spice and sweetness of the mind were in ample supply. We would discuss science and religion, music and the arts. I made her laugh, and she made me think more deeply about life's complexity. These online interactions would continue for quite some time before we would meet. There had been prior attempts at meeting for a drink or whatnot, but our schedules too often refused to synchronize. When the day finally did arrive wherein we could meet, I was broke as fuck, which only enhanced the anxiousness of meeting this utterly enchanting woman in whom I had already developed a permeating interest.

I had a few beers down the hatch before I even arrived. I arrived late. We had opted to meet at a brewery in Inglewood. My finances were tight so, after the Uber there, I had only enough for a couple rounds. Believing this would be just a short first meeting, I figured a couple pints each would be ample. It wouldn't be long until she footed the bill, and I was apologizing for being strapped for cash. She didn't seem too bothered by the fact at the time; after all, we were laughing and talking jovially away. The occasional moments of silence when we would make sudden eye contact, the inside jokes about hipsters and man-buns, and the energy I felt between us as we sat side by side at one of the long tables in the tasting room all felt natural and softly exhilarating. To gaze into her eyes, actually before me, was to forget the world at large.

The truth of our mutual interest was apparent and undeniable. The attempts of other men to redirect her interest fell flat and fruitless. For my part, I was only scarcely aware that anyone else was present at all. As the afternoon progressed into the hazy tone of early evening and we found ourselves tipsy and tantalized, she suggested I accompany her home. I was not expecting the invitation. In consideration of how her attractiveness in person had far exceeded expectation, I was beyond entertaining the notion of refusal. I was compelled.

We headed south into one of the more suburban areas of Calgary. The quiet streets, roundabouts, and cul-de-sacs of South Calgary seemed like a world apart to my mind, which was awash with craft beer and infatuation. Her home was dimly lit and welcoming. She left me alone on a sectional in the living room so she could change out of her work clothes. She smiled alluringly as she left the room. She returned in a matter of minutes, the quintessential little black dress draped across her slender form. The visual equivalent of a seductive whisper, she seemed to glide languidly through the room just outside of time itself. For the briefest moment, a heartbeat, it seemed as though she was poised in a tableau before my enraptured eyes. Just as I thought she could not be any more beautiful, she put on music. Early Dimmu Borgir filled the air with symphonic Norwegian black metal, and I was certain that before me was a woman even my most quixotic dreams would fail to imagine. As the thrill and enticement began to permeate my thoughts, so too did anxiety begin its maligned recital within.

The sensory intake was abundant. Bedazzled and impaired, I could feel the glitches tremble ever so slightly in the depths of my brain. I could feel myself becoming overwhelmed with stimuli. A sensation of something impending whispered in my skull as we embraced. Her lips on mine would then erase the world. Dopamine surged to squelch the flaring cortex. All would be well. Nestled together, we spoke softly and waited. There was a delivery forthcoming that was to enhance the night as it were.

I hadn't been there long before the night took a turn, swerving in a direction I hadn't intended. The small baggie that arrived provided just enough of a slick kick off-course as to render recovery and control fantastically beyond my reach.

What would then occur was a roller coaster, a cavalcade of emotional disruptions. I began a blathering display of instability. Covering the full gamut of unrestrained reactions, I was clearly unhinged. My spectrum of psychological and emotional instability in full glaring bloom, I indeed appeared to be off the rails. I interrupted with rambling nonsense and erupted into diatribes; her patience for me would wear thin. Incomplete thoughts forming broken sentences, I continuously misspoke and laboured fruitlessly to extract myself from a deepening pit of cognitive distress. My visible tears in response to her traumatic tale left her clearly questioning her decision to have invited me into her home. My failure to properly articulate the nature of my interactions with my drug-addled ex was greeted with disdain and distrust. Depersonalized and inebriated, I watched myself flail about in a very cerebral sense. She would pull away, justifiably so. I was not behaving in a manner that would warrant anything more than increased hesitation and disinterest. My outburst left me exhausted and I fell asleep on the sofa. She remained at the other end, awaiting daylight before requesting that I leave before her roommate got home. I slunk away, ashamed of my instability, and frustrated that my damaged and troubled brain had opted to careen out of control so unexpectedly and with such horrendous timing.

When I returned home, I messaged her to apologize for my discombobulated behaviour.

She would have none of it.

Accusations and condemnation were her general response. I struggled to plead my case. I likely made matters worse with my feeble attempts at explanation. So much is lost through text messages and the like that anything I had to contribute would have easily been perceived as excuses or worse. Regardless, I pressed onward, insisting that a misunderstanding had occurred and that the worst possible version of myself had coincidentally made itself known. It was during this exchange that I was informed that someone had told her I was a meth addict. I wasn't and am not, yet the malicious irony was not lost to me. I also begrudgingly accepted how believable such an assertion would be, considering my behaviour. At one point in our argumentative and disheartening exchange I stated flatly that I had issues with communication and emotion on account of my severe head trauma. Maybe she was responding to the message before that exact one when I read "Good luck finding someone that will put up with all that. You never will."

At the time, however, it cut to the quick and I instantly convinced myself she was right. After all, hadn't my brain damage previously brought stress, inconsistency, confusion, and frustration into past relationships? In one way or another, I was certain it had.

Had those words been spoken I would still hear the echoes as they resonated about my skull. There remains the same sense of unworthiness that has always been there, only now the tone and timbre contain something of the third person in them. I fully doubt that she had meant such harm. In the time I knew her there was an absolute lack of evidence that she could be that malicious, that insensitive. I had felt the kindness, the tenderness and the empathy that live within her and hadn't the faintest inkling of suspicion that she could be so cruel. Her intellect alone would remove her from such a lack of sympathetic understanding. Be that as it may, I had swallowed deeply the sentiment as I perceived it at the time. As it was a thought that had always lurked and sulked in the furrows of my mind, I assimilated it easily. The validity and affirmation of my lack of worth and value gave ample support to a long-held notion: it was better for everyone if I remained alone.

20

POPULAR DATING APP[REHENSION]

Over time, my unabated and persistent loneliness began to have the twitch and tick of paranoia, of self-deception. The notion of meeting anyone in a romantic sense had become a fanciful thought saddled heavily with maligning overtures of futility. I simply couldn't envision a circumstance wherein a woman would find meeting me to be a prelude to anything but disappointment and frustration. I had (and indeed have) so utterly convinced myself that my issues and struggles are unbearable that I couldn't imagine anything else to be true. Yet despite this, a timid voice could be heard adrift in the tempest of negativity. It insisted that the opposite was just as likely true and worth exploring.

    This damn pandemic having limited social venues and my social skills in tandem, I turned to a popular dating app to explore my options. I figured that if I could perhaps meet and connect with a stranger online, I could ease myself into societal normalcy again while simultaneously easing her into the latent issues that assail me, both factual and presumed. With thousands of women on the site, surely, I would match with one enough to get the ball rolling. Years ago, I had some minimal success in this approach, so I set about setting up my profile. I selected fun and whimsical photos to accompany my basic personal information. Yet after a couple of weeks of swiping this way and that, I had only garnered interest from four or five women, one of whom I believed was a bot developed by the site to make people feel noticed. After some adjustments to preferences and the like, nothing changed.

In retrospect, it was probably my opening line in the section on details—my tagline, if you like:

> Brain Damaged Man in His Forties
> Seeks Woman Out of His League
> To Ghost on Because of
> Social Anxiety

21
Memory Morphing to Mourning

Just over a week ago I was again on the Distress Hotline, a resource I use and recommend.

The strain and stress of navigating daily life had hit a disheartening and critical note. No, not a note. A cacophony of thoughts and feelings. With tears in my eyes and a nearly painful shortage of breath, I called in desperate panic. I delved into my issues. I delved into my history. The woman on the other end presented a concept I hadn't considered. She said I was grieving.

I spoke to her about my past life, about when it seemed all the simple triumphs were well in reach. I spoke of my current struggles. She brought them into tandem with the notion that I was grieving. I am. I am grieving the loss of the version of me I spent years cultivating and nurturing. The chef. The popular, charismatic guy. The happy and driving rebel that I identified with.

Fuck, I miss him.

Of course, I have had an earlier therapist explain the trick my mind has played on me. I researched the propensity for exaggerating the historic facts to our favour. So, as I don the bifocals of hindsight, besmirched by bias and the fog of egotistical self-preservation, I am clearly at a loss to capture the truth between varying perceptions of self. The erosion of the memories has hindered my understanding further. I know I have struggled for years, but to what extent? I would love to say I know who I am, especially considering how admirable my self-awareness is according to the medical community that supports me. I would love to be able to make the distinction between truth and ego driven conceptualization. I'd mostly love to equate.

When confronted with sudden challenges or in moments of stress there is by times a volta of depersonalization that occurs. It is a mere fraction of a second in duration and is only minutely acknowledged by my conscious mind. A solitary heartbeat when I am in stasis between two versions of self. The moment between the past and present is defined by nothingness. A sacred and disparaging place on the spectrum wherein I am neither my past nor present self. My memory of abilities and capacities from my life flash quickly before my mind's eye before being vanquished by the truth of my current hindrances. In that brief lacuna my actions are perceived as not my own. The desired responses are manifested in a muddied and haphazard way. The receding sense of a former self unable to maintain the reigns of control dissolves, leaving only a faint sentiment of something more. The self of the moment, the one that I am, always seems to fall slightly short of what was envisioned. Left with only the vague recollection of how this or that was once easier to manage, orchestrate and achieve, I suffer thorns and lashes of disillusionment and frustration.

Crestfallen and beleaguered, I ploughed forward. I knew full well that things could be worse. I do not, I can not allow myself to dwell on shortcomings and near misses. I owe gratitude to my good fortune that I can function at the level I do. I am thankful and remind myself every day of how much worse my life could be, all things considered. Though my job is not in the upper echelon of cuisine, I am able to work. Though my social circle has shrunk significantly, at least those that remain are dear. There are many positives that are present here within the tapestry of struggle and triumph, as can be said of anyone. Yet there is the notion that my life was, and could have been, more. More comfortable. More stable and secure. More imbued with successes and the accompanying accolades. More vibrant with confidence and vivacious with joy. More removed from even considering these notions at all.

As y memory was damaged, redacted, or destroyed by head trauma I cannot be certain of how it was before. Did I have the same degree of fear and worry that I now possess? If so, of what? How did it manifest? How did I cope with it? I do know with utter certainty that I managed it better then than I do now. Had it been worse, I doubt highly I would have made it this far. However, there is a chance that these spectres of my former self that wafted up from below on eddies of cerebral yearning are as much phantasms as ghosts from the past. Fantastic illusions dreamt to life by a faulty and desperate brain.

22
The Lies I Sire

The façade is real. It's tangible and visible. It's by times polished; by others, it's dingy. Through it, through the gaps and cracks, one can perceive the confusion, the turmoil it obscures. I can sometimes convince myself that nothing of the trauma seeps out; more often than not, it is quite the opposite. There is every reason to believe that others, particularly those that know, see my faults, my shortcomings. They may not be glaring but only faint, whisping eddies of the maelstrom I feel churning ceaselessly within me. Regardless, I strive to distract and deny the true nature of my predicament.

When asked how I am doing, if I'm OK, my habitual answer is "I'm well." Most days I *am* well, so the answer is true. Other days I use the token answer with a practised tone and delivery that so precisely match the sincere that I doubt anyone can discern the difference between an honest answer and the alternative. My projected self is thus no more than a fraudulent portrait painted painstakingly by the same hand and displayed under the low light of deflection. It's not just that I do not wish for someone to worry, nor is it as simple as not wanting to feel judged. It is more that if those two concepts were to coalesce, my suspicions would surely be confirmed, and concern born of judgement would warrant explanation. This would be difficult and draining.

As my obvious failures still stalk my every step, always behind and always breathing putrid air down my neck, I am all too aware that my situation must remain somewhat guarded. My early struggles after the most recent TBI still echo through dark chambers in my mind. The mistakes multiplied in those days, like bacteria left unchecked. I was never able to properly clear the residue and flare-ups are inevitable. The visage of the former self I have propped up before unassuming eyes being unattainable, I reinforce the façade with more tales of past exploits, former glories. I apply more thick brushstrokes, layered on in hope of sealing the cracks. Nothing dishonest—at the most maybe exaggerated for dramatic effect. A ruse of a tapestry meant to hide the discoloured wall behind it. I know I am not what I once was. I know that I am less than that man, but why should anyone else know? I keep others focused on, and entertained by, a past so far removed as to be a different life on a different world.

Thus, the charade is played out again and again. Inadvertently it often leads to failings and fumbles as I am unable to keep up the act. The paint starts to peel and chips fall away. The tapestry frays in time and I clamour for more flamboyant tones. I don't imagine anyone cares about it too damn much, though I do. My successes are so few and far flung that they can scarcely distract from my failures, my flaws for long. The edifice must remain unwavering for as long as possible. I must remain vigilant in my guardianship of what lies behind it, lest I be viewed and treated differently. Mistakes and misjudgements are akin to tiny deaths. The character, cultivated through necessity, dies, leaving only the actor alone under the lights and eyes.

Convincing others is a task, occasionally a daunting one. Commonly, however, it is easy, though not so easy as convincing myself. That trick seems to be as easy to perform as snapping one's fingers or combing one's hair. The seeds of self-deception were planted at a time long forgotten. That part of my mind that sows the seeds so intertwined with my more nurturing self that they appear as

Skull Fragments

one. An amorphous presence in my mind perpetually arguing with itself. Never knowing which has the upper hand, I succumb easily to either polarity. This results in a conundrum of sorts. Hopelessness is reinforced by the notion of hope, fear by the reality of fear. Doubt finds strength in the history of reasons to have had doubt. The confusion and frustration at my inability to understand leaves me exhausted as I try to determine whether I am indeed lying to myself or not. It is not the nature of reality or even my perception of it that has become untenable; it's my perseverance in pursuit of actuality that is dampened and lacklustre. I simple accept certain things as being true about my life, my condition. In doing so, it could be said that I have jilted a deeper purpose or stunted progress, I suppose. When struggles abound in all directions, is it not justifiable to take the easy way whenever you can? Seeing as what is true seems increasingly malleable depending on the information at hand, does it even matter at all?

My actions on that night in early January, though I would not change them, have set into motion a series of events from which the only escape I can fathom is delusion and deceit. Of course, this isn't applied in a blanketed manner over all aspects of my life, at least not to the same degree or for the same reasons. Sometimes it's a limbic go-to for flight from truth, rather than having to fight through another bout of emotional turmoil. Perhaps it is simply the dying embers of previous pride attempting a display of smoke and light in desperation for rekindling. Still again, it could be the cloak and dagger of shame that drive me into shadows behind the tapestry to stare at the discoloured wall.

When I'm left alone in my apartment, inebriated and without disruption, the veil has often been known to fall. The façade crumbles and I rage, weep, laugh, and sing, no rhyme or reason needed for any. That which is writhing within uncoils from itself, and polarities expunge unabashedly from me. My neighbours must think me properly mad. In those moments I couldn't care less. The deluge of emotion, stifled and incarcerated for days on end, spews forth in a fantastic and frantic display of honest liberation. I am not able to cower behind the folds as the tapestry flutters wildly on the gusts of tail winds begotten by such exuberant expulsion. The sadness and loneliness, the exasperation and the fear are gale-force propellants setting turbines in motion. Joy, relief, and hope begin to churn upward, milled into a permeating tincture. Mechanisms and remedies come to life, and I feel renewed. The cathartic consequence allots for the time and energy to refurbish the façade. A vision of steadfast strength and resilience again adorns the tapestry in vibrant shades.

Confined once more behind the shroud of distraction, I am again able to remove myself from those truths that would cause me such particular discomfort and those that perhaps would not, the former owing no regard to the latter, the latter's uncertainty succumbing to the former's likelihood. Failures and successes, fears and desires all subject to the same dimly lit perception, it does perplex me that one tends to garner any more attention than another. This is of no recourse, as it is far more essential that devotion be paid to maintaining the fabrication of the tapestry itself than exploring any alternatives. As much of my strength and perseverance, as perceived by others, are intrinsically part of that fabrication, I doubt it would serve me if I was to step out from between the tapestry and the discoloured wall.

23
Do the Things

On the inside of my bedroom door, tacked off-kilter with a ladybug pushpin, is a sheet of generic printer paper with the words "Do the Things" scribbled aggressively in black marker. A makeshift motivational poster designed to provide an interpretive directive to keep me at least marginally on track, it has hung there for years. A daily prodding, a gentle and insistent reminder that there *must be something* I can be doing to progress in my rehabilitation. The message lacks a specific determination, leaving it open to my own idealization, my own definition and interpretation of what should or could be accomplished. Just as long as something is done each day, no matter how slight, I can feel that progress has been made.

It also acts as an anchor of sorts, weighing me down so I don't allow my thoughts to become so fanciful as to lead my actions too far askew of obligations and responsibility. It has often been paired with a calendar posted on an adjacent wall that has more precise and pertinent information about what could, should, or must be done. That generic piece of printer paper with its simple and decisive message has been a cornerstone of my motivation and tenacity, though, admittedly I observe and acknowledge it less as time goes by.

Prior to that sheet of now off-white, with its scrawling black ink, I was familiar with the necessity of a calendar. The months after surgery were regimented by days on end of appointments. Therapy sessions at Sheldon Chumir were a near-daily constant, often two or three different therapists on any given day. In order to assure my attendance, I needed to keep a detailed account of when and with whom I would be meeting. When applicable, I would make note of subjects and issues that would pertain to the particular therapeutic encounter. Early on I was also required to track my obligations outside of the hospital: bill payments, EI report dates, therapeutic homework, and the like. The things I had to do. The most important was my steadfast attendance at my scheduled appointments. The visual reminder not only kept me punctual but gave me the encouragement to focus on forthcoming tasks. It was necessary for me to know if it was an occupational, psychological, or recreational session. The fore knowledge aided me in preparing for the tests and challenges associated with each respectively. I needed to be, and mostly was, diligent in duty as it pertained to my daily visits to the hospital near my home. I don't just mean that I had a 99 percent attendance, but that I was subsequently prepared to give 100 percent upon arrival with very few exceptions. I knew it was essential to do the work if I was to regain any semblance of the man I recalled being prior to my encephalitic incident.

 I'm assuming it was neuroplasticity at work. There I was reeling from the severe trauma of an epidermal hematoma after a three-on-one beatdown in which I was the one getting beat. My brain in traumatic disorder was malleable and likely yearning for reconstruction. So it was that the dopamine found its waterway into the ocean of growth potential. As my reliance on visual reminders became hardwired into my existence, I experienced the rewards for my labours. The dopamine cycle came into fruition as a result of the work I had done, which was fuel for the fire that empowered the work yet to come. The calendar would be filled with achievements, the tasks scratched off upon completion, the generic paper on my door reminding me not to rest on the laurels of those accomplishments.

The work continues. There are still things to be done. It's not always easy, either then or now. The days of static resolve and stagnant complacency are both behind me and on the horizon. I recall the day I left therapy as I just wasn't up to the challenge. I also remember doubling my efforts thereafter. The knowledge that there will undeniably be days wherein a simple sign on the back of a bedroom door will not suffice to motivate and encourage causes me little concern. A significant portion of the work is simply embracing and welcoming those days without letting them become a gyroscopic pivot point. The things that need, could, or should be done can wait long enough to catch your breath.

24

THERE'S A HOLE IN MY BUCKET

When I feel compelled to explain what it's like living with TBI at times of additional trouble or challenge, when my issues are similarly exaggerated, I now use this old folk song to attempt to communicate what I experience. I can't fetch the water to wet the stone, to sharpen the knife, to cut the straw, to plug the hole in the bucket I need to fetch the water. The song itself was presented to me as a child as an example of excuses and laziness. It has taken on new meaning and relevance now.

In the early days after the second of my craniotomies I struggled greatly. Retention of information was a challenge, as information and newly acquired knowledge would often seep away. I would grasp at straws of acuity and understanding with marginal success in an attempt to stem off that seepage, but seemed to lack the means and utility to do so to my satisfaction. The sharpness of wit and instinct which I once possessed had become dull and ineffective. I was not able to tailor a fix to problems with the same precession as I once could. Furthermore, I was hindered greatly when attempting to hone the skills to their previous efficiency. That laborious task seemed to be a dry and fruitless endeavour. Occasionally, this would result in frustration that I was not able to properly prepare or even understand the preparation fully. If only the knowledge could be retained, held fast and secure. If only the slow-draining insight would cease to escape from within that faulty vessel of cognizance, how much easier would it all have been?

That which needs repairing is the very thing that is required for the job. This troublesome conundrum can become a source of frustration and disheartenment. The task seems futile, and motivation is in diminishing supply. Thankfully, over time, I was able to realize that time was what I needed to solve the problem. I would approach the tedium of reverse-engineering the process or side-stepping the hurdles as needed. Essentially, a circuit breaker was required to disrupt the cycle. I'd consider the various steps as acutely as possible to determine which could be jury-rigged adequately to suffice a new starting point in a new cycle. It was a trial-and-error exercise that would occasion dutiful repetition to achieve desired ends.

The process renewed, by means of a makeshift contrivance, I would eventually find a solution, a means to proceed with tasks at hand. Though the interval of time may exceed expectations and preference, comforting confidence would be garnered through completion. As time passes, the skill required hones itself through tenacity and dedication.

25

THE ONGOING RECLAMATION

Shortly after the beat-down that hospitalized me and nearly ended my life, while I was still unable to work and attending therapy appointments daily, I strolled into my favourite bar, a popular barbecue joint in the downtown core of Calgary. I had been a regular there for years and had developed friendships with the staff. They were familiar with my situation. When I arrived, my friend was just finishing her shift, so we sat together to have a few drinks. We'd had many chats through the years and over the previous weeks she had become a dependable confidant regarding my traumatic experience. As we sat there, I felt compelled to thank her for all the support and understanding. She looked at me and smiled briefly before saying, "No. Thank *you*." She would go on to explain that any time she was having a bad day, was discouraged or unmotivated, she would think of what I was dealing with and had survived. My tenacity and stalwart devotion to overcoming my challenges were inspiring to her. We were smiling at each other with tears in our eyes before long.

In hindsight, that talk and others like it, were part of my motivation to write this. I wanted to share of my *self*, my struggles. Perhaps others could find understanding and encouragement, inspiration and strength. As much as writing this was therapeutic for me on a personal level, I hope it will benefit others. I would like to think there is a continuous hum, a tone that reverberates throughout—not just a single note, but a harmonious sounding of chords, the positive and negative chiming away in just such a way that one note scarcely begins to fade before another rises. I have, likewise, heard this song play as the score to the dozens of conversations I have had on brain injuries with people I have met through these years. The number of people affected—personally or by way of a loved one—is astounding. I hope by adding my voice those notes can be heard that much more clearly.

The positive of my more recent experience was the gift of knowledge and the tools to make my life, if not easier to navigate, at least easier to understand. The doctors, nurses, and therapists involved in my immediate recovery benevolently provided me with more than I can ever properly encapsulate. To them I express my perpetual and unyielding gratitude. Had only the medical community possessed the knowledge in my teens that they have now, how different would my life be?

That would be the other side of the coin. The knowledge I have now about the workings of the brain lends a breath of fevered air from time to time, fueling anger and resentment for the life with which I was saddled at fourteen. My thoughts that there is a chance that those years of confusion could have been different in some way do intervene upon my optimism and attitude often enough. I am well aware that it is hardly worth thinking about, as it cannot be changed. This understanding, however, can become elusive when I get introspective under unfavourable light.

There is obviously a lot of work left to do. To remain diligent and attentive to not just my needs, but to that which only hinders my progress. The struggle is ongoing. The challenges will persist until my final days. I won't always be vigorous in my efforts. I will stumble. I will fail. On occasion, I will, admittedly, not feel remotely like trying. For the most part, I truly believe I will continue to ride this wave on these uncharted waters.

From the beginning to now so much has changed.

About the Author

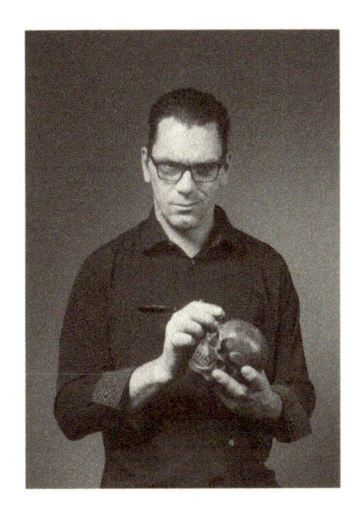

Len Roach has two traumatic brain injuries and at least a dozen concussions. By sharing his experiences, Roach hopes to help others better understand traumatic brain injuries and help people tell their own stories. *Skull Fragments: Expressions of My TBI Life* is his first book. Roach feels lucky to be able to write a book given that many survivors are unable to. He lives in Calgary, Alberta.